D1587504

DATE DUE

PRINTED IN U.S.A.

Choices in Palliative Care

Choices in Palliative Care

Issues in Health Care Delivery

Arthur E. Blank

Sean O'Mahony

Amy Selwyn

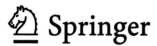 Springer

Arthur E. Blank, PhD
Assistant Professor
Co-Director
Division of Research
Department of Family and Social
   Medicine
Albert Einstein College of Medicine

Amy Selwyn
Medical Communications Services

Sean O'Mahony, MB, Bch, BAO
Medical Director
Palliative Care Service
Montefiore Medical Center
Assistant Professor
Albert Einstein College of Medicine

Library of Congress Control Number: 2007922359

ISBN: 978-0-387-70874-4   e-ISBN: 978-0-387-70875-1

Printed on acid-free paper.

9 8 7 6 5 4 3 2 1

springer.com

The book is dedicated to
K.S., and A.H.A. for Sean O'Mahony
M.A.K. and S.T.B. for Arthur E. Blank

Table of Contents

List of Contributors

Bob Arnold, MD,
Institute for Doctor-Patient Communication,
Section of Palliative Care and Medical Ethics,
University of Pittsburgh Medical School,
Pittsburgh, PA

Vikas Bhatara, MD,
Critical Care Medicine Fellow,
Montefiore Medical Center,
Bronx, NY

Arthur E. Blank, PhD,
Assistant Professor,
Co-Director
Division of Research,
Department of Family and Social Medicine,
Albert Einstein College of Medicine,
1300 Morris Park Avenue
Mazer 100, Bronx, NY

Carolyn Cassin, MPA,
Chief Executive Officer,
Continuum Hospice Care,
Jacob Perlow,
New York, NY

Alpana Chandra, MD,
Critical Care Medicine Fellow,
Montefiore Medical Center,
Bronx, NY

Andrea Cheville, MD,
Department of Rehabilitation Medicine,
Mayo Clinic
Rochester, MA

Martha Dale, MPH,
Executive Director,
Leeway, Inc.,
New Haven, CT

Linda Farber-Post, JD, BSN, MA,
Bioethicist and Clinical Ethics Consultant

Rita Fountain,
Coordinator, Pediatric Advanced Care Team,
Dana-Farber Cancer Institute and Children's Hospital,
Boston, MA

Nicole Fowler, PhD (c), MHSA,
Department of Medicine, Division of General Internal Medicine,
Section of Palliative Care and Medical Ethics,
Pittsburgh, PA

Randy Hebert, MD, MPH,
Department of Medicine, Division of General Internal Medicine,
Section of Palliative Care and Medical Ethics,
Pittsburgh, PA

Manoj Karwa, MD,
Critical Care Medicine Division,
Montefiore Medical Center,
Bronx, NY

Vivek Khemka, MB, BCh, BAO,
Palliative Care Fellow,
Palliative Care Service,
Montefiore Medical Center

Vladimir Kvetan, MD,
Montefiore Medical Center,
Division Chief,
Division of Critical Care Medicine,
Bronx, NY

Ruth Lagman, MD, MPH,
The Harry R. Horvitz Center for Palliative Medicine,
The Cleveland Clinic Foundation,
Cleveland, OH

Thierry LeJemtel, MD,
Department of Cardiology,
Tulane University School of Medicine,
Section of Cardiology,
Tulane, LA
Montefiore Medical Center,
Bronx, NY

Brenda Mamber, LCSW,
The Shira Ruskay Center,
Jewish Board of Family and Children's Services,
New York, NY

Franca Martino-Starvaggi, CSW,
Montefiore Medical Center, Palliative Care Service,
Department of Family and Social Medicine,
Bronx, NY

Ruth McCorkle, PhD, FAAN,
The Florence S. Wald Professor of Nursing,
Yale University School of Nursing,
New Haven, CT

Marlene McHugh, MS, RN, FNP,
Montefiore Medical Center, Palliative Care Service,
Department of Family and Medicine,
Bronx, NY

Adnan Mirza, MD,
Critical Care Medicine Fellow,
Montefiore Medical Center,
Bronx, NY

Sarah Myers, MPH,
Rand Corporation,
Arlington, VA

Sean O'Mahony, MB, BCh, BAO
Medical Director Palliative Care Service,
Montefiore Medical Center
Medical Director Jacob Perlow Hospice at Montefiore
Assistant Professor, Medicine and Family Medicine, Albert Einstein
College of Medicine
718-920-6378
F:718-881-6054

Linda Robinson, PhD, RNCS,
Associate Professor,
Hahn School of Nursing and Health Science,
University of San Diego,
San Diego, CA

Francine Rainone, PhD, DO, MS,
Montefiore Medical Center,
Department of Family and Social Medicine,
Bronx, NY

Jennifer Rhodes-Kropf, MD,
Division of Geriatric Medicine,
Department of Internal Medicine,
Montefiore Medical Center,
Albert Einstein College of Medicine,
Bronx, NY

Peter Selwyn, MD, MPH,
Montefiore Medical Center,
Albert Einstein College of Medicine,
Professor and Chairman,
Department of Family and Social Medicine,
Bronx, NY

Edmund H. Sonnenblick, MD,
Montefiore Medical Center of the Albert Einstein College of Medicine,
Bronx, NY

Tamara Vesel, MD,
Instructor in Pediatrics, Harvard Medical School,
Attending Physician, Pediatric Advanced Care Team,
Dana-Farber Cancer Institute & Children's Hospital,
Boston, MA

Declan Walsh, MSc, FACP, FRCP (Edin),
The Harry R. Horvitz Center for Palliative Medicine,
The Cleveland Clinic Foundation,
Cleveland, OH

Joanne Wolfe, MD, MPH,
Assistant Professor of Pediatrics, Harvard Medical School,
Director, Pediatric Advance Care Team,
Dana-Farber Cancer Institute & Children's Hospital,
Boston, MA

Preface

By 2050, 22% of patients are anticipated to live to be 85 years or older and expect to face 3 to 6 years of life with progressive disability (Fried, 2000). This increased longevity, evident in the United States and other industrialized societies, has to large extent been achieved through the technological advances of modern medicine and the development of health maintenance and preventive measures that are at least partially reimbursed for individuals with health care insurance. But as Fried noted, increased longevity comes with a price. More and more patients are living with the complications of chronic illnesses and toward the end-of-life, the patients, their caregivers, the providers involved with their care, as well as the institutions they may reside in, find themselves having to manage multiple physical, psychosocial, spiritual and emotional problems.

In the U.S., the multiple, chronic care needs faced by these patients and their caregivers are often ill served by fragmented systems of care. The current set of health care benefits in the U.S. are, for the most part, designed to meet the needs of patients with acute presentations of individual illnesses and enhance access to surgical and other interventions whose focus is on cure. In the face of payment streams that reward interventional, and single clinical problem oriented approaches to care, health care providers, organizations and payers struggle to create systems of care that can readily accommodate the multidimensional needs of end-of-life patients and their caregivers and support the demanding multidisciplinary team and or case management approaches needed to care for these patients.

As the evidence base that identifies unmet needs for patients approaching the end of their life accumulates and is reported in almost every healthcare setting (Teno, J.M. 2004; Emmanuel, E.J. 2000; Desbiens, N.A), new paradigms for palliative care medicine have emerged. These paradigms of care emphasize the importance of improved quality of life for these patients and their families, enhanced pain and symptom management, improved communication between providers, patients, and caregivers, and recognition of, and provision for, the multidimensional needs of the palliative care patients –needs that are psychosocial, spiritual, that involve greater coordination of medical and social services, and that offer bereavement services to caregivers after the patient's death. Such paradigms should be made available regardless of anticipated survival times for individuals with progressive chronic medical illnesses and their caregivers (Morrison & Meier, 2004).

In the first four chapters of this book, the contributing authors describe the complexity of clinical needs and barriers that currently exist to the provision of end-of-life care in different health care settings including homecare, acute care and long term residential care. The second set of chapters discuss palliative care in the context of dominant illnesses – Cancer, HIV/AIDS, Chronic Obstructive Lung Disease, Chronic Heart Failure, and Alzheimer's Disease. The next set of chapters focus around the complex needs of children and the elderly, and the last set of chapters address a broader set of issues: how to make the business case for palliative care, how to use Quality Improvement approaches to assess improvements being made in the provision of care, while the last chapter provides a framework for bioethical analyses and dispute mediation in the care of patients and caregivers at the end-of-life.

This book is the beginning of a journey that will need to be refined, and expanded as the American population becomes older as well as more culturally diverse. It is unclear, at this point, how those broad demographic shifts in American will shape the arguments in this book. It is our hope, however, that these arguments will become clearer and that remedies to the fragmented care provided to patients can be found.

All of our contributors have been concerned with improving the care of patients and their caregivers, and we are indebted to each for the time and effort they have put into producing their chapters. They have explored the evidence base for end-of-life care in their individual professional areas and each provided valuable insights which we, and they, hope will result in improved palliative care.

We would like to thank Bill Tucker and his staff at Springer Press for their advice, support and patience in completion of this book. We'd also like to thank Ronit Fallek for helping us manage the initial phases of this book. Lastly each of would like to thank our own caregivers who suffered mightly with us as we edited and lived with this text. Arthur wants to thank Margaret for the time lost, the sacrifices, and her constant encouragement. Sean would like to thank Sean, Kathrina and Howard for their advice, insights and support.

References

Fried, L.P. (2002). Epidemiology of aging. *Epidemiology Rev.* 22(1):95-106.

Lunney, J.R., Lynn, J., Foley, D.J., Lipson, S., Guralnik, J. (2003). Patterns of functional decline at the end of life. *Journal of the American Medical Association.* 289(18):2387-92.

Teno, J.M., Weitzen, S., Fennell, M.L., Mor, V. (2001) Dying trajectory in the last year of life: does cancer trajectory fit other diseases? *Journal of Palliative Medicine.* 4(4):457-64.

Teno, J.M., Claridge, B.R., Casey, V., Welch, L.C., Wetle, T., Shield, R. (2004). Family perspectives on end-of-life care at the last place of care. *Journal of the American Medical Association.* 291(1): 88-93.

Emanuel, E.J., Fairclough, D.L., Slutsman, J., Emanuel, L.L. (2000). Understanding economic and other burdens of terminal illness: the experience of patients and their caregivers. *Annals of Internal Medicine.* 132(6):451-459.

Desbiens, N.A., Mueller-Rizner, N., Connors, A.F., Jr., Wenger, N.S., & Lynn, J. (1999). The symptom burden of seriously ill hospitalized patients. SUPPORT Investigators. Study to understand prognoses and preferences for outcome and risks of treatment. *Journal of Pain and Symptom Management.* 17(4): 248-255.

Morrison, R.S., & Meier, D.E. (2004). Clinical practice. Palliative care. *New England Journal of Medicine.* 350 (25): 2582-2590.

1
Palliative Care in Acute Care Hospitals

Randy Hebert MD MPH*, Nicole Fowler PhD MHSA, and Robert Arnold MD

1. Introduction

Changes in the demographics and healthcare needs of the U.S. population have forced a shift in the types of healthcare services that people want and need. Hospitals are faced with the challenge of meeting the needs of an increasingly older and frailer population. An American born in 2000 can expect to live to nearly 77 years old; a 65 years old can expect to live another 18 years (Federal interagency forum on aging-related statistics, 2002). In addition, technological advancements have allowed individuals to live longer with chronic, advanced illness. For example, the elderly often experience chronic, progressive diseases that they will live with for three to six years before death (Fried, 2000). These changes have placed pressures on the healthcare system to design practices and programs that best meet the needs of the population. Table 1.1. highlights some of the demographic and care needs that hospitals must address.

Because the last years of life are often characterized by physical and psychological distress, greater demands on family caregivers, and increased needs for external support, there is a growing need for palliative care services. Palliative care programs are often staffed by an interdisciplinary team of physicians, nurses, social workers, counselors, and clergy (the composition of which is often contingent on the program's funding source and practice setting) and is focused on the relief of the physical, psychological, and spiritual suffering of patients with life-threatening illness, and their families. The increasing number of hospital-based palliative care programs is evidence of the demand for these

RANDY HEBERT • NICOLE FOWLER • ROBERT ARNOLD • Division of General Internal Medicine, Section of Palliative Care and Medical Ethics, MUH 933W 200 Lothrop Street, University of Pittsburgh School of Medicine, Pennsylvania 15213, USA and *Corresponding author: Assistant Professor of Medicine, Division of General Medicine, Section of Palliative Care and Medical Ethics, MUH 933W, 200 Lothrop Street, Pittsburgh PA 15213, Phone: 412-692-4258, fax: 412-692-4315, e-mail: hebertrs@msx.upmc.edu

TABLE 1.1. U.S. Healthcare demographics

The median age of death is greater than 75 years and will increase
The proportion of the population older than 85 years old will double to 10 million by 2030
90% of Americans die after living for a time with one or more chronic, life-threatening illness
98% of Medicare decedents spent and spend at least some time in a hospital in the year prior
    to death
53% of all deaths occur in hospitals
15-65% of all decedents have at least one stay in an intensive care unit (ICU) in the six months
    prior to death

Source: Federal Interagency Forum on Aging-Related Statistics. www.agingstats.gov
Centers for Medicare and Medicaid Services. www.cms.hhs.gov

TABLE 1.2. The population of patients for whom palliative care is appropriate

Those with life-threatening illness where cure or reversibility is a realistic goal (e.g. stroke)
    but the illness causes significant burden
Those with chronic, life-limiting conditions (e.g. chronic heart or renal failure)
Those with a terminal condition, whether the result of a chronic or acute illness or event,
    who are unlikely to recover and for whom palliative care is the predominant goal

services—15% of hospitals and at least 26% of U.S. academic teaching hospitals have a palliative care consult service or an inpatient unit (Billings & Pantilat, 2001; White *et al.*, 2002).

Table 1.2 highlights the diverse patients who may be served by palliative care; the criteria are based on symptoms and the complexity of needs rather than on age or stage of disease (National Consensus Project, 2004a).

In this chapter we will present information that should be helpful to a prospective hospital-based palliative care program director and to the administration of health care organizations. First we will summarize the arguments about the need for and benefits provided by palliative care programs. We will then present information on the planning, implementation, and evaluation steps necessary to ensure that a palliative care program meets the needs of the hospital in which it operates, the clinicians who care for patients, and the patients and families living with illness.

2. Why Palliative Care in Acute Care Hospitals?

First, hospitals are where the most severely ill patients are found. It is estimated that 12% of acute care patients are appropriate for palliative care services (Edmonds *et al.*, 2000). Unfortunately, the care of hospitalized patients with serious, advanced illness is often characterized by the under-treatment of symptoms, conflicts about who should make decisions about the patient's care, impairments in caregivers' physical and psychological health, and depletion of family resources (Desbiens *et al.*, 1999; Emanuel *et al.*, 2000). Palliative care aims to improve the quality of life for these patients and their families by managing pain and symptoms, maintaining communication, providing psychosocial, spiritual, and bereavement support, and coordinating a variety of medical and social services (Morrison & Meier, 2004).

Second, hospitals are where most expenditures occur. Nearly all Medicare beneficiaries spend some time in the hospital during the last year of life and roughly 25% of Medicare dollars are spent on patients in the last 60 days of life. In addition, the 63% of Medicare patients with greater than two chronic medical conditions account for 95% of Medicare costs (Lubitz & Riley, 1993). Palliative care programs can help provide quality care that is fiscally responsible by preventing unnecessary or unwanted medical interventions (Raftery *et al.*, 1996; Smith *et al.*, 2003).

Third, hospitals are the place where transitions in care often occur. Because of the many healthcare providers involved, there is potential for miscommunication. For example, patients at end of life often have long hospital stays and are typically cared for by multiple physicians, each with an opinion on what is best for the patient. Two hallmarks of palliative care, communication and coordination of care, are necessary to ensure that patients and families receive patient-centered care and have smooth transitions from the hospital to home, nursing home, or hospice (de Haes & Koedoot, 2003; Parry *et al.*, 2003).

3. What are the Benefits of Palliative Care in Acute Care Hospitals?

By meeting the needs of an increasingly aging population with multiple chronic illnesses, palliative care programs can provide several potential benefits to acute care hospitals. These include:

3.1. Lower Costs

Although the data on the cost-effectiveness of palliative care is mixed, there are several ways in which palliative care programs may lower costs (Payne *et al.*, 2002). First, by helping to transition patients appropriately to care settings with lower acuity, palliative care programs may help reduce length of stay and intensive care unit (ICU) utilization (Miller & Fins, 1996; Raftery *et al.*, 1996). Transfer of such patients out of the ICU also allows for more acute care and elective admissions, appropriate use of critical care beds, and reduced number of hours that the emergency department must be placed on "diversion." Second, palliative care can help minimize the utilization of unwanted high intensity interventions as well as unnecessary and often painful or ineffective tests and medicines (Fins *et al.*, 1999). By helping to initiate discussions about resuscitation and treatment goals, palliative care programs can appropriately divert resources being used from patients away from expensive and intense life-prolonging therapies to less expensive comfort orientated and supportive therapies (Campbell & Guzman, 2004). Finally, by improving communication and coordination of care between clinicians, patients, and families, palliative care programs can provide high quality care while lowering ancillary costs (Hoffmann, 1998).

3.2. Improved Pain and Symptom Management

A cornerstone of palliative care is that patients do not suffer from uncontrolled symptoms. Successful approaches to the assessment and management of pain and other symptoms have been established in clinical trials (Higginson *et al.*, 2003). For example, 85% to 95% of terminally ill patients' pain can be relieved with oral regimens that are not dose limited by troublesome side effects (Doyle *et al.*, 2004). Not only is symptom control important for the patient, improved symptom control is associated with better well-being in the surviving family members (Valdimarsdottir *et al.*, 2002).

3.3. Providing Support to the Primary Team

Many clinicians have difficulty providing good end-of-life care (Christ & Sormanti, 1999; Norris *et al.*, 2004; Sivesind *et al.*, 2003; Sullivan *et al.*, 2003). Until recently, there has been little training in palliative care for health care providers. Palliative care services can support the clinicians responsible for the care of the patient by:

By providing expertise in pain and symptom management.

Helping to facilitate communication about goals of care between patients, families, and healthcare providers.

Helping to coordinate care by providing a liaison between the primary service and the other healthcare providers involved in the patient's care.

Educating clinicians about the role of hospital-based palliative care and enhancing their skills through role modeling and case-based teaching.

Despite these justifications for hospital-based palliative care programs, most hospitals do not have a program and struggle to develop new programs. In an era of high health care costs and slim profit margins, if new programs are to be developed, implemented and sustained, they need to serve the needs of hospitals in which they are based and demonstrate improved outcomes. In the next section, we will review the crucial elements to creating support and gathering the necessary information to design, market, implement, and evaluate a new hospital-based palliative care program.

4. Conducting a Needs Assessment

The first step in developing a palliative care program is to conduct a needs assessment (Table 1.3). Palliative care is not a solo practice. Strong collaborative and team-building skills are critical for success. Successful leaders will have the skills to collaborate with the multiple stakeholders–administrative, clinical, and community–whose ongoing support is necessary to the integration and sustainability of the program.

The following section describes the different components of the needs assessment and discusses the process by which the information is gathered and used in program planning and implementation.

4.1. Systems Assessment

A commitment from stakeholders throughout the hospital will be necessary to influence the culture of acute care hospitals to accept a palliative care program. Many program developers assume that educating hospital staff about the benefits of palliative care is sufficient to generate support. The planning team, however, needs to refocus the traditional ideas of "selling" palliative care and use the assessment of the stakeholders to help them shape and design the program. Find out what the stakeholders want from a program and then tailor the program to meet these needs. The assessment will also help determine what outcomes will be important to the stakeholders. For example, it is important to meet with the hospital's administrators and its financial planning and billing managers to determine how they think palliative care services can benefit the hospital–is it in reducing costs, meeting Joint Commission on Accreditation of Healthcare Organizations (JCAHO) compliance standards regarding symptom control, generating good public relations, etc?

TABLE 1.3. Purposes of a needs assessment

To reconcile the priorities of palliative care proponents with those of the hospital administration, clinicians, patients, and families, and with the existence of similar or overlapping services in the community

To ensure that the palliative care program meets the needs of its consumers and is accepted as an integral part of the hospital continuum of patient care

To establish baseline information that will be necessary when attempting to evaluate outcomes

To provide insight into the design of the program, staffing needs, and clinical focus e.g. ICU patients vs. outpatients, symptom management vs. care planning, etc.

To allow program developers to address the common misperceptions that clinicians have about palliative care, *before* launching the program

These include the view that:

Palliative care teams "take over" the care of the patient at the expense of the primary team

Palliative care teams encourage patients and families to "give up" rather than to continue with aggressive care

Palliative care is a form of healthcare rationing.

4.2. Clinical Assessment

Proponents of palliative care can easily identify clinical units or populations that they believe need their services; they tend to view palliative care in terms of the benefits that it can provide to patients. While these benefits are important, a key to generating support for a new program is to view clinicians as the primary consumers of the program. According to the Center to Advance Palliative Care, marketing the benefits of palliative care to potential consumers (physicians, nurses, social workers, care managers, clergy etc.) is not nearly as effective in gathering support as is stressing how palliative care can help them (Meier & Sieger, 2004). Clinicians will only utilize the services of the palliative program to the extent that they perceive the services to be of use to them. The clinical assessment will allow the program to focus on providing services that clinicians want, whether it is help with pain and symptom management, time-intensive communication with patients and families, or care plan coordination. Without the support of clinicians, who will be the major source of patient referrals, a palliative care program will fail, regardless of the expected benefits it may bring. Of course, individuals interested in developing a palliative care program must be mindful to promise only what is deliverable and sustainable within the constraints of existing and likely resources.

Physicians, nurses, social workers, and other care providers are likely to have different needs. It is important to discern what issues they struggle with in caring for seriously ill patients before attempting to convince them that a palliative care program can help. For example, physicians may be primarily interested in help with difficult to manage symptoms or having an experienced team available to talk with patients and families about goals of care. Nurses may be most interested in a service that helps to facilitate communication between the multiple members of the healthcare team. Social workers may want help with coordination of care issues, especially as related to discharge from hospital to home, nursing home, or hospice. Surveys, in-depth interviews with key leaders, or focus groups can be used to obtain this information.

4.3. Population and Community Assessment

Another step in designing a program is to use the information obtained from the system and clinical assessment to describe the types of patients who will benefit from the services. Gathering data on projected needs and volumes will enable the palliative care planning team to determine the program model that best fits the hospital's needs and resources and to establish baseline data that will be necessary for assessing program effectiveness. Consider some of the following questions:

How large is the *target population* that you intend to serve? How many patients died in a given year? Where did people die? How many people were referred to hospice?

What *hospital departments* could most benefit from palliative care services—critical care, oncology, geriatrics, cardiology, surgery etc? The populations served by these departments are different. For example, patients and families in an intensive care unit may be most in need of improved communication about goals of care whereas oncology outpatients may benefit most from better pain control. In addition, the associated healthcare providers may have different opinions on the role palliative care should play in the care of their patients. Will they use palliative care services primarily to manage symptoms, discuss end-of-life issues, coordinate care and disposition, etc?

A next step is to identify and evaluate the community resources that provide palliative care services or that deliver care for patients with chronic disease. These may include hospices, nursing homes, pain clinics, or home health services. Information that should be gathered would include:

1. The number and type of services that are available,
2. Their reputation among patients and clinicians,
3. Their ability to satisfy the community's need for palliative care.

This step is essential for identifying gaps in currently provided services and for determining how a proposed palliative care program might help fill these gaps. In addition, this step can help form partnerships with community providers who can enhance the quality of the hospital-based program by providing continuity of care to patients discharged from the hospital and potentially providing another funding stream.

4.4. Financial Assessment

In an environment of limited health care dollars, a palliative care program needs to demonstrate that it can improve clinical outcomes, at a cost at least comparable to conventional care (Bruera & Suarez-Almazor, 1998). Medicare, a fixed rate (capitated) system, is the primary payment mechanism for hospitalized patients. Payment is based on the Diagnostic Related Group (DRG) (Davis *et al.*, 2002). The DRG, however, was developed for acute illness and is a poor method for stratifying illness severity and resource utilization in palliative care. For example, it does not take into account special circumstances like progressive disease, co-morbidity, or psychosocial issues, all of which prolong hospitalization (Rutledge & Osler, 1998). Because of the limitations of the DRG, case-mix indexing (CMI) is usually necessary to ensure that cost and resource use comparisons are equitable for palliative care programs versus other hospital services (Davis *et al.*, 2001). The CMI is a DRG with a relative weight scale based on resource, labor, and supply utilization. CMI indirectly reflects illness severity and better predicts cost of care as compared to a DRG.

Understanding your patient population, payer mix, and utilization rates for certain services is important for assessing the potential financial impact of a new palliative care program. For example, if administrators reveal that the readmission rates for Medicare beneficiaries admitted under DRG 127 (heart failure and shock) is the most costly or preventable expense to the institution, the palliative care program may want to focus on that high-risk group. To the extent possible, it will also be helpful to demonstrate costs to the hospital (in length of stay and ancillary expenses) for failing to identify and institute appropriate services and discharge options for this population. Many hospitals already have a methodology for tracking the impact of quality added services (e.g. the value of social work or care management) to the bottom line. In addition, state Department of Health data can provide useful information on length of stay for patients in local peer institutions with and without palliative care programs. This data will allow for benchmarking within the institution and local region. Finally, it is important to quantify and document the value-added revenues that will result from the program. These may include:

Increased patient and family satisfaction
Improvements in pain and symptom management
Reduction in length of stay
Reduction in unnecessary and costly interventions and procedures
Appropriate referrals to affiliate or hospital owned hospices, home care or
    nursing home services

5. Developing a Business Plan

In a cost conscious environment, new projects must be carefully planned and evaluated to ensure clinical as well as economic success. As the needs assessment is being conducted, there is a need to create a business plan that combines information from the needs assessment with prospective program outcomes. The business plan (Cohn & Schwartz, 2002):

Reassures the hospital administration that a palliative care service is needed
    and that program development is being approached in a fiscally responsible manner
Is a demonstration of the planning that went into program development
Defines the range of services to be offered in light of the stated program goals
Serves as a tool for performance appraisal

A business plan should include the following components (Meier & Sieger, 2004):

5.1. Justification

The justification summarizes the rational for a palliative care program, presents the medical and social context for the proposed program, and includes data from the needs assessment. National, regional, and local data about other palliative care programs and about the demographics of the hospital service area can be included.

The justification is where the following questions are answered:

How will a palliative care program help the hospital meet its goals?
How will a palliative care program meet the needs of physicians, nurses, social
   workers, clergy, etc.?
What services will the program provide?
What model will the program adopt and why?
How will the program be fiscally viable?

5.2. Program Goals

Program goals will be dictated by the information gathered during the needs
assessment. Program success will be measured in part by the ability of the program to meet feasible and specific goals agreed upon by the palliative care team,
hospital administrators, physicians, nurses, social workers, and other hospital
consumers. Depending on the needs assessment, potential goals may include the
following short term (e.g. 12 months) and longer-term (e.g. 3-5 years) goals:

Clinical outcomes: e.g. symptom burden, quality of life, clinician satisfaction,
patient and family satisfaction, etc.

Demographic and utilization statistics: e.g. Number of consultations and
percentage of patients with particular DRGs who receive services from the
palliative care program, percent of palliative care patients who died in the hospital, length of stay for patients before and after palliative care intervention,
hospice referral rates, etc.

Fiscal statistics: e.g. Number of ICU days saved as a result of palliative care,
number of procedures (e.g. surgery, hemodialysis, etc.) avoided as a result of
palliative care, emergency department utilization and readmission rate after the
index palliative care consult, revenue generated from inpatient hospice patients,
emergency department utilization, and readmission rate post index consult.

5.3. Delivery Model

There is no "right" program model. Rather, the model must fit the needs,
resources (hospital size, bed availability, availability of trained palliative care
staff, etc.) and culture of each institution. For example, if your hospital is an
academic hospital familiar with the involvement of physician consultants, a
physician-centered palliative care consult service may be the best fit. On the
contrary, if your hospital is a community hospital with a voluntary medical
staff that follows patients in various settings (e.g. the hospital, outpatient clinics, long term care facilities), a nurse or social worker-led model with strong
involvement from a community hospice may work best. The advantages and
disadvantages of the various delivery models are:

Consultation service: A consultation service is typically staffed by physicians,
advance practice nurses, or social workers, who see patients throughout the
hospital.

Advantage: This is a good mechanism for introducing palliative care to clinicians as it reaches the largest number of geographically separated healthcare providers. This model also requires very little overhead costs. Although paid work time can be much higher for a physician, the salary of an advance practice nurse with the requisite skill set often approximates that of a physician. In addition, in our experience, advance practice nurses need significant training/experience prior to being able to function independently. Moreover, physicians are often more comfortable caring for patients with complex medical problems. However unlike with physician consultants, a nurse or social worker palliative care consultant does not require a formal consultation order to see patients. Therefore, nonphysician and family requests for palliative care can easily be accommodated.

Disadvantage: Hospital staff may not be comfortable with palliative care, may be unaware of when to ask for palliative care consultation, and may be uneasy with certain recommendations e.g. using opioids for dyspnea. As a result, the willingness to implement recommendations or accept a consultation may vary by discipline of the consultant. Also, the palliative care team may not have their recommendations followed as they serve only as consultants to the primary physicians. Additionally, a formal order for a palliative care consult must be written in the clinical chart in order for physicians, nurse practitioners, or physician assistants to bill the patient's insurance for their services. If the program is dependent on clinical revenue, it may take several months for the program to generate the revenue necessary to support the palliative care clinicians' time.

Inpatient Unit: Palliative care patients are clustered together in a section of the hospital or in designated beds.

Advantage: The hospital staff on that unit quickly becomes skilled in palliative care. The concentration of staff allows for the palliative care staff to educate the other healthcare providers. Additionally, the culture and philosophy of care in a specific unit or designated beds within a unit may be more conducive to the philosophy of palliative care. Patients and families would have easier access to a different array of disciplines (music therapy, massage therapy, etc.) and feel more supported in their decision to choose a palliative plan of care.

Disadvantage: Geographic concentration deprives staff and patients from other parts of the hospital of the benefits of palliative care. The number of patients cared for by the palliative care program is limited to the number of beds in the unit. The physical separation of palliative care patients from other hospital patients may deepen the belief of some physicians, nurses, patients, and families that palliative is an "all or nothing" choice. Financially, inpatient units have higher overhead costs than consultation models. Although, financial drain is less of a factor if length of stay is carefully managed and if the institution has a high capacity with frequent admissions.

Combined consultation and inpatient unit:

Advantage: Allows concentration of staff expertise and can enhance continuity of care in the hospital.

Disadvantage: Availability of trained staff for both unit and the consult service.

Outpatient palliative care clinic:

Advantage: Provides the greatest continuity of care for patients discharged from the hospital. Also provides a valuable resource to physicians caring for patients with multiple physical and psychosocial symptoms but who are not so ill that they need to be admitted to the hospital.

Disadvantage: Not available to hospitalized patients. In addition, seriously ill patients may not want to or may have difficulty following up with both the palliative care service and their primary physician. Debilitated patients who rely on family caregivers to travel to and from clinic may have particular difficulty. Another disadvantage is that outpatient palliative care visits can be time intensive. Physician payment for outpatient services is often insufficient to sustain a clinic on clinical revenue alone.

Given these advantages and disadvantages, an important factor to keep in mind when developing a program is that different models of care delivery will be needed to meet the needs of different types of palliative care patients. Integrated programs that focus on how best to meet the needs of diverse palliative care patients are often the most successful and sustainable.

5.4. Marketing

Marketing is often perceived as a one-time effort that takes place early in the life of a program. In fact, it begins during the needs assessment and should be a continuous, seamless part of program development, implementation, and sustainability. Hillestad and Berkowitz wrote that "marketing is the process of molding the organization to the market, rather than convincing the market that the organization provides what they need" (Hillestad & Berkowitz, 1984). Marketing efforts, therefore, must be continually reviewed and revised as needed based on the needs of the hospital administration, partnering organizations, clinicians, patients, and families. Otherwise, the program may find its support base decreasing.

5.5. Operations Plans

The operations plan is a list of resources required to put the new program into operation and a description of how the program will function:

Administrative and clinical staff: This is the most important component of the operations plan (Vetter *et al.*, 2001). Ideally, the team members should be named and their experience and expertise described. If a position is vacant, the operations plan should describe the education and experience necessary to fill the position and when, how, and where the program will recruit the necessary staff.

Data and financial systems: The plan should outline the type of data that will be collected on a regular basis and how it will be collected and analyzed. Additionally, the plans should include how professional fees will be coded, entered, and submitted to the payer. This often happens at the physician practice level, but the hospital-based palliative care team should be aware of the process and know whom to work with to ensure that the clinician's time is being covered.

Administrative and clinical space: The dimensions, the timetable for readying the space, and any constraints on the use of the space should be described.

Equipment and supplies:

Medicine formulary: Program developers need to ensure that medicines that are commonly used in palliative care (e.g. methadone, hycosamine) are available and stocked in the necessary pharmacies.

Clinical pathways: These may include symptom assessment and control protocols, sedation policies, and transfer policies. A good source for information on symptom, communication, and coordination protocols is the National Consensus Project (National Consensus Project, 2004b).

Quality assurance: This section should address quality and safety measures. Methods for measuring and improving outcomes should be outlined.

5.6. Financial Plan

This part of the business plan must establish an accurate range of financial parameters that support the proposed program's viability. For hospital administrators, the financial plan may be the most important component of the business plan. The financial plan should include a short term (12 month) and long-term (3-5 year) budget of revenues, cost savings, and expenses based on volume and program growth assumptions.

Development of a financial plan begins with a list of sources of revenue from payers including Medicare, Medicaid, and commercial insurers, as well as fund-raising activities and philanthropy. In addition, revenue generated by the hospital for inpatient hospice patients can also be included if the palliative care program plans to utilize inpatient hospice care.

While the revenue streams may be limited for hospital palliative care programs under the current financing structure, the financial plan should include estimations of cost savings as a result of palliative care interventions. For example, if data obtained from the needs assessment reveals that long lengths of stay in the ICU are causing a financial drain, estimates about palliative care penetration in the ICU and about the cost per day of ICU care can be used to calculate savings resulting from decreased lengths of stay.

Typical expenses for a palliative care program include salaries and benefits, rent, taxes, equipment, etc. (Tarantion, 2001). Because financial operations involve tax and accounting considerations, cash management strategies, and financial reporting, this section should be prepared with the aid of financial specialists within the hospital. After identification of the marketing and operations-related costs and estimating the anticipated program revenues, it becomes possible to judge whether the revenue stream is adequate to support a new program. Finally, the financial plan should include contingency plans if the assumptions about program revenue, cost savings, and expenses do not hold. A long-term plan for financial sustainability is particularly necessary if the major funding sources for the program include unreliable sources such as hospital and medial school funding or philanthropy.

5.7. Implementation Plan

The implementation plan ties together the entire business plan and assures the hospital administration that the palliative care program will be delivered as promised. The plan describes potential problems and how they will be addressed. A timetable provides a visual landmark for the proposed activities and identifies important milestones e.g. recruiting and hiring of key faculty, the addition of services.

The business plan is not a static document. Rather it is a fluid process that will undergo a number of revisions as the program matures and the palliative care leadership meets with administrators, key clinicians, and potential donors. Regular meetings with the different members of the palliative care team will also ensure that the business plan is continually updated to reflect the current environment.

6. Sustaining a Palliative Care Program

6.1. Measuring Outcomes

How will the success of the program be measured? The success of a new program depends on the ability to demonstrate results. Baseline measurements, clinical and financial, should be established prior to launching the program and systems must be in place to track the effects of the program on those measurements over time. Tracking and reporting outcomes demonstrates accountability, keeps hospital administration and clinicians abreast of the positive effects of the palliative care program, and allows the palliative care team to make adjustments to the program as needed.

Monitoring outcomes will depend on data collected from patients and families, clinicians, medical records, and hospital databases. Important outcome measures include:

Patient data: Patient characteristics (e.g. date of consult, gender, ethnicity, religion), DRG/ICD9 code, functional status, number of patients seen, lengths of stay prior to and after being seen by the palliative care program, percent of patients discharged alive, discharge location, the percentage of inpatient deaths for patients with DRGs that are often seen in palliative care, and referrals to hospice are examples of data that may be important to track based on the program's goals.

Clinical data: Advance care planning, pain and symptom assessment at defined intervals, and patient and family satisfaction are important clinical data to collect.

Financial data: Costs per day before and after palliative care consultation, length of stay in the hospital and ICU before and after palliative care consultation, and unwanted or unnecessary procedures, medicines and treatments avoided as a result of the palliative care intervention are examples of possible financial data that could be tracked and analyzed. If possible, much of this data should be collected in patients seen by the palliative care service and in control groups with equivalent length of stay, CMIs, or DRGs.

6.2. *Managing Growth*

As the program matures and the hospital administration, clinicians, patients, and families become more knowledgeable about palliative care and the benefits that it can bring, the program will grow. Plans should be in place to adjust the delivery model and the composition and number of staff, depending on program growth because clinicians will stop referring patients if the program does not have the capacity to meet their needs. Issues to consider include the:

Hospital environment: Have there been changes in hospital services that may compete or complement palliative care services (e.g. a new pain program, an ethics consultation service, a multi-disciplinary geriatrics program)? Are there new administrative champions or opponents of palliative care?

Financial environment: What has been the financial impact of the program? Does the value added justify the addition of new resources (e.g. more clinical staff and space)?

Clinical environment: Is the number of referrals increasing, decreasing, or remaining stable? Is the CMI/patient acuity changing? Is the program seeing patients earlier in their hospital stay or disease process? How do clinicians hear about the program? Who is referring to the program? How could the program reach those clinicians or departments that do not make use of the palliative care services?

Program directors should also periodically assess the palliative care staff. How is their morale? Are their signs of burnout? As the program grows, new policies that help prevent staff burnout may need to be instituted for things such as weekend coverage or vacation time. Directors should also ensure that the staff has opportunities for professional development and advancement. These issues have implications for staff turnover (Baumrucker, 2002).

Community environment: Are there new referral sources outside the hospital? Are there competing services in the community (e.g. a new hospice program)?

In revisiting the business plan, the palliative care team may need to make changes to the delivery model, number and composition of the clinical staff, budget, or marketing plan.

References

Baumrucker, S. J. (2002). Palliative care, burnout, and the pursuit of happiness. *Am Journal of Hospice and Palliative Care, 19*(3), 154-156.

Billings, J. A. & Pantilat, S. (2001). Survey of palliative care programs in United States teaching hospitals. *Journal of Palliative Medicine, 4*(3), 309-314.

Bruera, E. & Suarez-Almazor, M. (1998). Cost effectiveness in palliative care. *Palliative Medicine, 12*(5), 315-316.

Campbell, M. L. & Guzman, J. A. (2004). A proactive approach to improve end-of-life care in a medical intensive care unit for patients with terminal dementia. *Critical Care Medicine, 32*(9), 1839-1843.

Christ, G. H. & Sormanti, M. (1999). Advancing social work practice in end-of-life care. *Social Work in Health Care, 30*(2), 81-99.

Cohn, K. H. & Schwartz, R. W. (2002). Business plan writing for physicians. *American Journal of Surgery, 184*(2), 114-120.

Davis, M. P., Walsh, D., Nelson, K., Konrad, D., & LeGrand, S. B. (2001). The business of palliative medicine: management metrics for an acute-care inpatient unit. *American Journal of Hospice and Palliative Care, 18*(1), 26-29.

Davis, M. P., Walsh, D., Nelson, K. A., Konrad, D., LeGrand, S. B., & Rybicki, L. (2002). The business of palliative medicine–Part 2: The economics of acute inpatient palliative medicine. *American Journal of Hospice and Palliative Care, 19*(2), 89-95.

de Haes, H., & Koedoot, N. (2003). Patient centered decision making in palliative cancer treatment: a world of paradoxes. *Patient Education and Counseling, 50*(1), 43-49.

Desbiens, N. A., Mueller-Rizner, N., Connors, A. F., Jr., Wenger, N. S., & Lynn, J. (1999). The symptom burden of seriously ill hospitalized patients. SUPPORT Investigators. Study to Understand Prognoses and Preferences for Outcome and Risks of Treatment. *Journal of Pain and Symptom Management, 17*(4), 248-255.

Doyle, D., Hanks, G., & Cherny, N. (2004). *Oxford Textbook of Palliative Medicine. 3rd ed.* Oxford, England: Oxford University Press.

Edmonds, P., Karlsen, S., & Addington-Hall, J. (2000). Palliative care needs of hospital inpatients. *Palliative Medicine, 14*(3), 227-228.

Emanuel, E. J., Fairclough, D. L., Slutsman, J., & Emanuel, L. L. (2000). Understanding economic and other burdens of terminal illness: the experience of patients and their caregivers. *Annals of Internal Medicine, 132*(6), 451-459.

Federal interagency forum on aging-related statistics, Older Americans 2000: Key Indicators of Well-Being (2000). Table 12A. "Deaths: Final data for 2000," National Vital Statistics Reports. www.agingstats.gov. Retrieved November 7, 2004.

Fins, J. J., Miller, F. G., Acres, C. A., Bacchetta, M. D., Huzzard, L. L., & Rapkin, B. D. (1999). End-of-life decision-making in the hospital: current practice and future prospects. *Journal of Pain and Symptom Management, 17*(1), 6-15.

Fried, L. P. (2000). Epidemiology of aging. *Epidemiological Reviews, 22*(1), 95-106.

Higginson, I. J., Finlay, I. G., Goodwin, D. M., Hood, K., Edwards, A. G., & Cook, A. (2003). Is there evidence that palliative care teams alter end-of-life experiences of patients and their caregivers? *Journal of Pain and Symptom Management, 25*(2), 150-168.

Hillestad, G. G. & Berkowitz, E. N. (1984). In *Health care marketing plans: From strategy to action* (pp. 35-36). Homewood, IL: Dow Jones-Irwin.

Hoffmann, D. E. (1998). Pain management and palliative care in the era of managed care: issues for health insurers. *Journal of Law, Medicine and Ethics, 26*(4), 267-289, 262.

Lubitz, J. D. & Riley, G. F. (1993). Trends in Medicare payments in the last year of life. *New England Journal of Medicine, 328*(15), 1092-1096.

Meier, D. E. & Sieger, C. E. (2004). *A Guide to Building a Hospital-Based Palliative Care Program*. New York: Center to Advance Palliative Care.

Miller, F. G. & Fins, J. J. (1996). A proposal to restructure hospital care for dying patients. *New England Journal of Medicine, 334*(26), 1740-1742.

Morrison, R. S. & Meier, D. E. (2004). Clinical practice. Palliative care. *New England Journal of Medicine, 350*(25), 2582-2590.

National Consensus Project. www.nationalconsensusproject.org (2004a). Retrieved November 7, 2004.

National Consensus Project. Clinical Practice Guidelines for Quality Palliative Care. www.nationalconsensusproject.org/guidelines (2004b). Retrieved November 7, 2004.

Norris, K., Strohmaier, G., Asp, C., & Byock, I. (2004). Spiritual care at the end of life. Some clergy lack training in end-of-life care. *Health Prog, 85*(4), 34-39, 58.

Parry, C., Coleman, E. A., Smith, J. D., Frank, J., & Kramer, A. M. (2003). The care transitions intervention: a patient-centered approach to ensuring effective transfers between sites of geriatric care. *Home Health Care Service Quarterly, 22*(3), 1-17.

Payne, S. K., Coyne, P., & Smith, T. J. (2002). The health economics of palliative care. *Oncology (Huntingt), 16*(6), 801-808; discussion 808, 811-802.

Raftery, J. P., Addington-Hall, J. M., MacDonald, L. D., Anderson, H. R., Bland, J. M., Chamberlain, J., & Freeling P. (1996). A randomized controlled trial of the cost-effectiveness of a district co-ordinating service for terminally ill cancer patients. *Palliative Medicine, 10*(2), 151-161.

Rutledge, R., & Osler, T. (1998). The ICD-9-based illness severity score: a new model that outperforms both DRG and APR-DRG as predictors of survival and resource utilization. *Journal of Trauma, 45*(4), 791-799.

Sivesind, D., Parker, P. A., Cohen, L., Demoor, C., Bumbaugh, M., Throckmorton, T.,Volker, D.L., and Baile, W.F. (2003). Communicating with patients in cancer care; what areas do nurses find most challenging? *Journal of Cancer Education, 18*(4), 202-209.

Smith, T. J., Coyne, P., Cassel, B., Penberthy, L., Hopson, A., & Hager, M. A. (2003). A high-volume specialist palliative care unit and team may reduce in-hospital end-of-life care costs. *Journal of Palliative Medicine, 6*(5), 699-705.

Sullivan, A. M., Lakoma, M. D., & Block, S. D. (2003). The status of medical education in end-of-life care: a national report. *Journal of General Internal Medicine, 18*(9), 685-695.

Tarantion, D. P. (2001). Understanding financial statements. *Physician Executives, 27*(5), 72-76.

Valdimarsdottir, U., Helgason, A. R., Furst, C. J., Adolfsson, J., & Steineck, G. (2002). The unrecognised cost of cancer patients' unrelieved symptoms:a nationwide follow-up of their surviving partners. *Britain Journal of Cancer, 86*(10), 1540-1545.

Vetter, L. P., Carden, R., & Wilkinson, D. S. (2001). Strategic planning in a clinical environment. *Clinical Leadership Management Reviews, 15*(1), 34-38.

White, K. R., Cochran, C. E., & Patel, U. B. (2002). Hospital provision of end-of-life services: who, what, and where? *Medical Care, 40*(1), 17-25.

2
Palliative Care in Nursing Facilities

Brenda Mamber LCSW

November 15, 2004

Mrs. Serrano is an 83 year old resident of a Nursing Home. She has been widowed for many years and has lived in the Nursing Home for the past 5 years. Mrs. Serrano has multiple chronic illnesses' which contribute to her weakness and her inability to care for herself. She also exhibits mild dementia. Her primary caretakers in the facility, the Certified Nurses Aides (CNAs) generally describe her as "someone who wants to be left alone", additionally describing her as "hostile and agitated". The CNAs had reported Mrs. Serrano's behavior to the facility nurses. But given that for most of the day Mrs. Serrano appeared calm, further assessment did not appear warranted by the staff. Among her caretakers, Mrs. Serrano became known as a "problem resident", one to be avoided as much as possible.

The CNAs who were assigned to Mrs. Serrano provided her personal care (i.e. bathing, dressing, and transferring) with competence, all the while enduring the daily targeted screaming, cursing, and agitation. "Mrs. Serrano is just mean" was the explanation most often offered by the CNAs.

Unfortunately the scenario described, is not an isolated one. Residents and nursing home caretakers are engaged in similar situations every day. Additionally, we know that 25% of all elderly nursing home residents with pain receive no analgesia, with the oldest and cognitively impaired resident more at risk. The SAGE study group of 4003 elderly nursing home residents demonstrated a correlation between under medication of pain and advanced age (Bernabei *et al.*, 1998). It is widely acknowledged that care in nursing homes *must* change (Orloff-Kaplan *et al.*, 2000), and that the experience of providing the care must improve, if we are going to have the resources to care for our growing aging population. This chapter highlights a number of issues related to current trends in palliative care in Nursing Facilities, including: sample research projects, palliative care curricula and training programs, and program services. A model of Palliative care will be described that is designed to meet the comfort needs of long-term care residents, and improve the quality of the work experience of the nursing home staff.

BRENDA MAMBER, LCSW • The Shira Ruskay Center/Jewish Board of Family and Children's Services, New York, NY.

Current practice has, in almost all palliative care programs, connected the application of palliative care to terminal illness (as in hospice), or to life-threatening/life limiting illness (as in hospital based palliative care programs). The current application of palliative care philosophy, practices, and services in long-term care nursing facilities has followed suit with a policy of providing palliative care to long-term care patients who are facing either terminal illness, or life-threatening illness. In an effort to expand the application of care to patients who do not fall within the Medicare Hospice six-month terminal prognosis eligibility criteria, new evaluative tools need to be designed. To determine if a resident might be appropriate for palliative care services, many facilities have, in addition to their standard assessment, adopted the use of a question, "Would you be surprised if the resident died in the next year?" (Johnson *et al.*, 2003). The question is an effort to establish additional palliative care criteria which will allow for the inclusion of residents whose diagnoses have historically proven to be difficult to prognosticate. Clearly however, the resident's eligibility for palliative care still remains within a framework of terminal to life-limiting illness. The need to widen our view of palliative care beyond end-of-life, the need to improve care to all long-term care residents, and the need to provide all nursing home staff (particularly CNAs) with additional skills and enhanced meaning is essential as we face the challenge of an aging population.

1. Current Projects

- *The Jewish Home and Hospital Life Care System of New York* co-sponsored their first palliative care conference in November 2002. Among others, John Carter and Eileen Chichin presented on the palliative care program that they developed within the Jewish Home facility. Adopting a Physician/Nurse consultation model, Carter and Chichin (2003) rely on referrals and are primarily caring for residents at end-of-life (63% having a prognosis of less than 3 months).

Some of the challenges that Carter and Chichin (2003) noted in providing palliative care in a facility are:

- Misconceptions about palliative care in general
- Difficulties associated with assessing discomfort in cognitively impaired residents
- The majority of hands-on-care is delivered by paraprofessionals
- Financial support
- Reimbursement Issues
- Fears about Regulatory Oversight

Carter's and Chichin's (2003) recommendations for the integration of palliative care in nursing homes include:

- Obtaining administrative buy-in
- Starting with a small, interested team
- Providing the team with basic and advanced education
- Starting small and then extending palliative care throughout facility
- Developing a hospice contract

In 2001, Tuch and Strumpf (*Genesis ElderCare and University of Pennsylvania School of Nursing*) initiated research activities focused on education, and the creation of a palliative care team in each of the six nursing homes participating in the study. While their model aimed to integrate palliative care into the mainstream of the nursing home care, the focus of the intervention was on life threatening illness and end-of-life care. Tuch and Strumpf employed a full-time palliative care nurse coordinator as part of the project. She divided her time between all sites, and was essential to the success of the project.

Tuch and Strumpf (2002) identified these challenges:

- Turnover in leadership staff
- Limited involvement from physicians
- Limited number of professional nurses
- Turnover in clinical staff
- Time-stressed staff who were reluctant to take on new tasks
- Perceived incompatibility between regulatory standards and palliative care

In a summary of their findings Tuch and Strumpf (2002) recommended the following as key components to improving palliative care in the nursing home:

- Committed leadership (Director of nursing, administration, corporate)
- Operational and clinical teams
- Palliative care consultation and on-going support
- Involved medical directors and primary care physicians
- Integration of palliative care principles in critical processes
- Regulatory over site
- Reimbursement
- Culture change

In response to the Partnership for Caring/The Fan Fox and Leslie R. Samuels Foundation background paper on "Moving Palliative care Upstream: Integrating Curing and Caring Paradigms in Long Term Care" (Orloff-Kaplan *et al.*, 2000) a number of initiatives were developed in New York City. The Metropolitan Jewish Health System developed a study that evaluated the impact of an experimental educational model. The study focused on changing nursing home staff attitudes and knowledge about palliative care, and effectuating positive changes in practice outcomes such that the delivery of palliative care is moved "upstream" in the disease/treatment trajectory (Kyriacou and Nidetz, 2002). Findings, as reported by Kyriacou and Nidetz (2002), suggest that continuous training in palliative care may improve receptivity and confidence in the provision of palliative care. The project attempted to broaden the vision of palliative care, applying the care and principles to the larger chronically ill nursing home population. The trainings were provided to staff from 2 nursing homes, but notably missing from the training program were CNA's.

In 2000, the Labor Management Project of the 1199 Hospital League Health Care Industry Planning and Placement Fund, Inc. also responded to the Partnership for Caring/The Fan Fox and Leslie R. Samuels Foundation background paper to upstream palliative care in nursing homes. In an unpublished grant request, the goal of this 2-year project was to explore how a palliative care approach could be introduced in a nursing home for all long-term care residents (e.g. upstreaming palliative care). The primary intervention included a 20-week palliative care curriculum that targeted CNA's as the participants. Unfortunately, there were inadequate design processes for a meaningful evaluation of the impact of the training on the quality of care for the residents under the care of the participants. Additionally, there were no institutional plans established to reinforce the palliative care education upon completion of the training sessions, nor were institutional changes made to encourage the utilization of new skill sets. In the unpublished final report to The Fan Fox and Leslie R. Samuels Foundation it was reported that within the scope of educating CNA's in regard to the concepts of palliative care, the training was successful (Mamber, 2002). Unfortunately in addressing the more global goal of improving the care to all long-term care residents though the participation of the CNAs in the palliative care course, the success of the project has not been evidenced.

2. Models of Care

In palliative care in Nursing Homes, Steps for Success: A Guide to Developing a Quality Palliative care Program, Rosendahl-Masella et al. (2004) report the findings of their survey to evaluate palliative care services in New York City nursing homes. They identify the following highlights from their research:

• 97.3% of the facilities participating in the study indicated that they provide some form of palliative care service.

While:

• 37% of the facilities did not have written palliative care policies.
• 61% of the facilities did not have a formal written definition of palliative care.
• More than 5% of the patients in the majority of the facilities were estimated as receiving palliative care

These statistics demonstrate a clear need for a uniform education among nursing home administrators and staff about the full range and goal of services under palliative care. "As noted, relatively few facilities have a "true" palliative care program and, even in the model programs, 66.7% estimated that less than 15% of their patients were receiving palliative care" (Rosendahl-Masella *et al.*, 2004).

In the nursing homes that were surveyed, Rosendahl-Masella *et al.* (2004) report that 59% had contracts with hospice programs. While palliative treatment plans are at the core of hospice services, having a hospice program for your residents is not synonymous with having a palliative care program. The most common palliative care model evidenced was the scatter bed consultation model. In this model the nursing facility has identified staff that work together to provide palliative care and institute palliative care treatment plans for referred patients who reside throughout the facility. Even within this model there is a wide variation, anywhere from 1-10 staff members. All or most of those team members usually have additional responsibilities within the facility beyond palliative care. CNAs are almost never identified as part of the palliative care team. Some programs have established relationships with hospital based palliative care experts (Bronx Community Palliative Care Network presentation, 2003) for medical consultation, while other programs rely on their internal expertise. These programs generally target residents at end-of-life, or those with unmanaged severe pain syndromes associated with life-limiting illnesses.

The institutional challenges to this model is the difficultly of appropriate identification and referrals of residents to the palliative care team (Carter and Chichin, 2003). It relies on the often, untrained staff throughout the facility to astutely assess the need and appropriately access the palliative care team. The staff that comprises the palliative care team are often limited and/or over extended in their overall responsibilities. Additionally, there may be a challenge (e.g. staff skill sets, resources, cultural resistance) in instituting an individual palliative care treatment plan, which may be contrary to customary procedures, in the context of a large facility. Most of the consultation model programs are sponsored by philanthropy which threatens the long term program viability.

Another model of palliative care utilized within facilities is the designated unit or cluster bed model. The facility designates a specific area or entire unit for the care of residents who are coming to the end of life. Some nursing facilities contract with hospice programs for in-patient hospice care and utilize a unit for both in-patient hospice care and nursing home resident palliative care. While this model usually provides a more comprehensive team approach from the entire unit staff, it still faces some challenges when addressing the needs of the larger nursing home population. By the very nature of the designated bed design, the utilization and provision of palliative care becomes limited to the specific numbers that can access the designated beds. By targeting those units/beds for palliative care, the palliative care focus in the institutional is potentially narrowed, both in the criteria that are established for residents to receive palliative care (end-of-life, life threatening) and in the number of residents that can access the service.

It is widely acknowledged that the development of palliative care programs and teams necessitate specific education of facility staff. Palliative care education appears to be focused in two directions. In their book Improving Nursing Home Care of the Dying: A Training Manual for Nursing Home Staff, Henderson *et al.* (2003) provide us with an excellent training program and curriculum for all staff of a nursing home. In particular, it is noted that their training curriculum is designed for multidisciplinary participation, noting the significant contribution/responsibility of the CNA in providing care. However, from a broader perspective of palliative care, the limitation of this training program is its narrow focus on caring for the dying.

In their training manual, Performance Based Palliative Care in the Nursing Home: Closing the Gap Between "Knowing" and "Practicing", Kyriacou *et al.* (2003) created an educational program to focus on the palliative care needs of chronically ill patients as well as patients at the end-of-life. The education program however has a limited focus on professional nursing facility staff, and is not inclusive of CNA staff.

3. Looking to the Future

The current trends to increase palliative care to residents in nursing homes are limited in scope. The focus on increasing contractual agreements with hospices, instituting limited and focused palliative care programs, units, services within facilities, and the development of external consultative relationships are positive moves, but remain limited due to the focus on end-of-life care.

Today 1.6 million people reside in the 18,000 nursing homes in the United States. In the year 1999, 777,500 deaths occurred in nursing homes, which represented approximately 25% of all deaths in the U.S. (The National Nursing Home Survey, 1999). The average length of nursing home residence for those who died in these institutions was two years, compared with the 2.38 year average length of residence for all nursing home admissions (NNHS, 1999). These figures clearly tell us that the vast majority of residents admitted to nursing homes are severely ill. Due to Medicare hospice regulations, those residents would largely not be certified as terminally ill (six month or less prognosis), and would therefore be ineligible for hospice care for 75% of their stay in a facility. Only 1% of the total nursing home population is enrolled in hospice at any given time (Petrisek and Mor, 1999). It seems clear that the integration of palliative care for all long-term care patients should be initiated at the time of the nursing home admission and follow them through discharge or death.

For nursing home residents, the ability to define the point when a disease, or more often, multiple diseases, become "life-threatening" in the context of terminal illness, has historically proven to be a barrier to patients receiving hospice care (Zerzan *et al.*, 2000). Nursing homes are, and will continue to be, institutions that provide care beyond the rigid constraints of in-patient hospitalization criteria. Most of their residents have needs that exceed the services available through traditional home care programs, and have diagnoses or prognoses that fall outside the eligibility framework for hospice care. It is a disservice to our growing nursing home population to continue to apply the standard definitions of palliative care (used in hospice and/or hospital based palliative care programs) to the initiation of palliative care services in nursing homes.

In New York City there are limited statistics available representing the number of residents enrolled in palliative care programs? Nor are there evaluative studies for the majority of these programs. These statistics clearly represent what we in health care already know; there is a huge gap between the need, and the care that is provided to residents who are living their last months and years of life in nursing homes.

Current health policy and reimbursement structures discourage use of palliative care and hospice care for nursing home residents. Quality standards and reimbursement rules provide incentives for restorative care and technologically intensive treatments rather than labor-intensive palliative care. Reimbursement incentives and fears about adherence to state and federal regulations also limit its use (Zerzan et al., 2000).

In a 1997 national survey, 56% of all nursing home days were paid by Medicaid. Medicare paid for approximately 15%, with the remaining days paid privately or by other sources (NNHS, 1997). The national average per diem rate was $105. / Medicaid, and $213. / for Medicare. In New York City, the per diem rates are approximately double for both the Medicaid and Medicare payment rates. These figures clearly demonstrate the challenges that nursing home administrators face when on average in New York City, 80% of the daily resident billable days are paid by Medicaid. In our current sluggish economy, the need to maximize new admissions to nursing home beds with residents who are eligible for Medicare reimbursement is a daily priority.

The Medicare benefit also allows a nursing home to bill Medicare when a resident is admitted following an acute hospitalization (three day minimum). This Medicare annual benefit is for a maximum of 100 days, assuming a documented skilled nursing need is identified. For the long-term care resident (those not admitted for restorative rehabilitation or sub-acute level of care) this reimbursement structure proves to be a financial disincentive for nursing homes to minimize their discharges to hospitals, or to incorporate specialized services that could provide expert pain control and/or symptom management. Under the current Medicare/Medicaid reimbursement structure there is no increased benefit to compensate nursing homes for providing enhanced symptom management, specialized pain control, nor palliative care. Additionally, the hospice nursing home Medicaid "pass through payment system" is complex and frequently misunderstood by nursing home administrators. The contract created between a hospice and a nursing home rarely takes full advantage of the financial (and otherwise) incentives that are allowed under New York State regulations. A resident, who is electing hospice care, would by regulation utilize Medicare for the hospice payment and Medicaid for the nursing home room and board payment. In this situation the nursing home would not have any potential to capture the Medicare reimbursement rate during the life of the resident. These financial and regulatory issues, have often proved to create barriers and/or underutilization of hospice care within the nursing home. With fiscal concerns becoming more and more a matter of daily survival for nursing homes; and the regulatory systems providing disincentives for the integration of hospice and palliative care in nursing homes; the question of who will take care of our sick elderly, and how will they take care of them must be addressed.

4. Nursing Home Staffing

In 1997 (National Nursing Home Survey) there were 1.4 million nursing home staff, more than 950,000 of whom were nursing staff. Certified Nursing Assistants (CNAs) held about 65% of all positions.

CNAs provide approximately 80-90% of all care. The job of the CNA can be difficult and strenuous.

In the Senate hearing of the Special Committee on Aging (July 2002), research was presented on the first part of a nursing home staffing study that Congress mandated in 1990. The initial findings include:

Nationwide, more than half – 54%- of nursing homes are below the suggested minimum staffing level for nursing aides. These aides are the lowest paid and least trained of all nursing home staff.

Nearly one in four nursing homes – 23%- was below the suggested minimum staffing level for total licensed staff.

Nearly one-third – 31%- were below the suggested minimum staffing level for registered nurses, which is 12 minutes per patient per day.

The report concluded that low staffing levels contribute to an increase in severe bedsores, malnutrition, and dehydration, which lead to increased hospitalization.

High turnover in nursing home staff, currently at 40% to 75% nationally, and as high as 100% in certain facilities, make it difficult to attract, train, and re-train an adequate workforce (Cohen-Mansfield, 1997). Low wages, lack of advancement opportunities, difficult work environments, competing entry level positions all contribute to high turnover rates among CNAs.

Current research has identified a number of additional issues that could positively impact CNA retention. Not surprisingly, economic conditions play a significant role in staff retention. However, management communication and staff empowerment also contribute significantly to staff satisfaction and retention. The ability to have a meaningful, respectful, and outcome directed exchange with managers is a significant part of the CNA feeling valued in their employment (Banaszak-Holl and Himes, 1996). Additionally, Banaszak-Holl and Himes found that in nursing homes where CNAs participated in care planning meetings, the staff turnover rate was 50% below other facilities (1996).

It is essential that palliative care educational programs target this group. But CNA palliative care education is not enough. Nursing home administrators and managers must embrace a broader definition of palliative care as a philosophy of care, and integrate a palliative care model of care for all long-term care nursing home residents, not just those facing the end-of-life. Institutional changes, and policies and procedures need to change to support new staff learning and skills. However slowly, the cultural environment of nursing homes must shift to begin to reflect the growing needs of not only our aging population, but of the population of workers who will be the care providers. A palliative care environment can provide a framework by which palliative care is integrated into all resident care plans from the time of admission, does not necessitate a terminal prognosis, and invites all staff to inform the quality of life of each resident.

"Mrs. Serrano is just mean" was the explanation most often offered by the CNAs.

How much care in nursing homes is provided in the context of . . . "that's the way we've always done things"? With the best of intentions, the suffering of residents, like Ms. Serrano can easily go unnoticed or unresolved. Ms. Serrano does not have a terminal illness, nor would she be expected to die within one year. She is certainly not eligible for hospice care, nor would she be included in most nursing home palliative care programs. The current cultural climate within nursing homes does not necessarily look at a resident's quality of life, outside of end-of-life, if at all. It is difficult for new nursing home staff, or even seasoned staff to begin to look at things in a new light. Understanding suffering and its relationship to behavior can have a tremendous impact on the quality of life of the residents, and the quality of life of the staff in providing care.

5. Creating a Nursing Home Palliative Care Environment

The conceptualization that palliative care, inclusive but not limited to end-of-life care, is applicable to all residents facing the challenge of chronic, debilitating illness is a core foundation of this paradigm. The paradigm of creating a nursing home palliative care environment will offer the nursing home staff both a philosophical framework and a delivery system by which to achieve these goals for all long-term residents in their care.

The main objectives and goals of the paradigm are to:

Improve the quality of life/comfort of all long term care residents through the application of medical, psychological, social and spiritual interventions consistent with palliative care and to integrate a new palliative care model into the traditional operational care delivery system of nursing facilities. Some of the elements involved in the changed system would be to:

1. Educate all nursing home staff, residents, and families in the philosophy and practices of palliative care, applicable to all residents in long term care (chronic illness and life- threatening illness).
2. Engage all newly admitted resident's in a palliative care assessment.
3. Create effective interdisciplinary care teams for resident centered care.
4. Integrate problem-based care planning within current practice.
5. Engage CNA staff in the continuous care planning of residents.
6. Incorporate system for direct report between CNA shifts on each resident.
7. Increase utilization of hospice services for enhanced end-of-life resident care and on-going staff education.

The nursing home palliative environment is a model of a delivery system that can be integrated into existing long term care delivery systems, and can be modified to meet the needs of specific institutions. The main underpinning of the paradigm is the conceptualization of palliative care as comfort care. Instituting a nursing home palliative care environment is not in conflict with curative or restorative care. Creating a palliative care environment is a compliment and an enhancement to all care provided in nursing homes, and although focusing the caregiver on the quality of life of the resident, does not alter the medical treatment goals of the resident. The care plan of the individual resident may continue to focus on the restorative or curative aspects of care, or may be "comfort" only. The manner in which the care is provided, utilizing palliative care philosophy and practice is a key to the potential for all residents to achieve the optimum quality of life.

6. Conclusion

Long-term care facilities are growing, residents are sicker, and the care provided is more complicated than ever. Nursing home staffs are working harder, administrators are working with less and less resources, and yet many nursing homes maintain their priority to provide the best possible care to all residents. Customer service and culture change initiatives in nursing homes are all part of a movement to improve care. The palliative care movement, first through the integration and delivery of hospice programs, but most recently through palliative care consultation models, is slowly making its way into mainstream nursing home care. Currently 25% of all deaths in the United States occur in nursing homes. If through our current efforts in hospice and palliative care in nursing homes, we are able to improve the quality of life for 777,500 individuals yearly (The National Nursing Home Survey, 1999) the palliative care movement in nursing homes would be a huge success. But is it enough? The 1.6 million (and growing) residents of nursing homes, and the significant numbers of their caretakers all need a better environment to live, to work, and ultimately to die. As noted, there are many barriers to the establishment of palliative care programs. Beyond philanthropic support, the funding for the development of programs has been limited. It is time for CMS and state legislators to revise the current Medicare and Medicaid reimbursement systems to allow for additional spending for comfort and care of our most vulnerable and fragile population. It is time to broaden our concept of palliative care, to be inclusive of all patients in long-term care. It is time to create palliative care nursing home environments as places to live which embrace hospice and end-of-life care, but also focus on quality of care for all residents and their caretakers.

References

Aviv, M., Jackson, J.G., Cox, K., & Miskella, C. (1999). Evaluation of project providing community palliative care support to nursing homes. Health & Social Care in the Community, 7(1):32-38.

Banaszak-Holl, J., & Himes, M.A. (1996). Factors associated with nursing home staff turnover. *The Gerontologist*, 36:512-517.

Berger, A. (2001). Palliative care in long-term care facilities: A comprehensive model. *Journal of the American Geriatric Society*, 49(11):1570-1.

Bernabei, R., Gambassi, G., Lapane, K., et al., for the SAGE Study (1998). Management of pain in elderly patients with cancer: Systematic assessment of geriatric drug via epidemiology. *Journal of the American Medical Association*, 299, 1877-9.

Carter, J.M. & Chichin, E. (2003). Palliative care in the nursing home. Oxford University Press, Washington, D.C.

Chichin, E.R., Burack, O.R., Olsen, E., & Likourezos, A. (2000). End-of-life ethics and the nursing assistant. New York: Springer Publishing Co.

Cohen-Mansfield, J., Ejaz, F., & Werner, P. (2000). Satisfaction surveys in long-term care. New York: Springer.

Ersek, M., Kraybill, B.M., & Hansberry, J. (1999). Investigating the educational needs of licensed nursing staff and certified nursing assistants in nursing homes regarding end-of-life care. *American Journal of Hospice & Palliative care*, 16(4): 573-582.

Ersek, M. & Wilson, S.A. (2003). The challenges and opportunities in providing end-of-life care in nursing homes. *Journal of Palliative Medicine*, 6(1):45-57.

Ferrell, B.A. (1995). Pain evaluation and management in the nursing home. *Annals of Internal Medicine*. 123(9):681-7.

Ferrell, B.A., Ferrell, B.R., & Rivera, L. (1995). Pain in cognitively impaired nursing home patients. *Journal of Pain and Symptom Management*, 10(8): 591-598.

Froggatt, K.A. (2001). Palliative care and nursing homes: Where next? Palliative Medicine, 15(1):48.

Gorman, M.P. (2003), Presentation: Bronx Community Palliative care Initiative, Palliative care in Nursing Homes, Schervier Nurisng Care Center Conference, New York City.

Hanson, L.C., (2003). Creating excellent palliative care in nursing homes. *Journal of Palliative Medicine*, 6(1):7-9.

Henderson, M.L., Hanson, L.C., & Reynolds, K.S. (2003). Improving nursing home care of the dying: A training manual for nursing home staff. New York: Spring Publishing Co.

Innovations in End-of-Life Care (2001). Special thematic issues: Promoting better pain management in long-term care facilities. 31(1). Available at: www.edc.org/lastacts

Johnson, D.C., Kutner, J.S., & Armstrong, J.D. (2003). Would you be surprised if this patient died? Preliminary exploration of the first and second year patients' approach to care decisions in critically ill patients. BMC Palliative care, 2, 1 of 9 pages. Available at www.biomedcentral.com.

Joint Commission Website (2004). Available at: <http://www.jointcommission.org>

Keay, T.J. (2002). Issues of loss and grief in long-term care facilities. In K.J. Doka (Ed.), Living with grief: Loss in later life. Hospice Foundation of America. Keay: Washington, DC.

Kyriacou, C.K., Hirschman, K.B., & Henry, M.R. (2003). Performance based palliative care in the nursing home: Closing the gap between "knowing" and "practicing". *Journal of Palliative Medicine*, 5(5):757-758.

Last Acts Palliative care Task Force (1997). Lasts acts. Care and caring at the end of life. Precepts of Palliative care. Available at: www.lastacts.org/docs/profprecepts.pdf

Levine, K.M. (2000). The circle of care: Establishing a palliative care service in a long-term care facility. *American Journal of Hospice and Palliative care*, 17(4):222-223.

Mamber, B., The Labor Management Project of the 1199 Hospital League Health Care Industry Planning and Placement Fund, Inc. (2002). Upstreaming Palliative care. Unpublished Final Report Partnership for Caring/The Fan Fox and Leslie R. Samuels Foundation.

Mezey, M.D., Bottrell, M., Mitty, E., Ramsy, G., Post, L.F., & Hill, T. (2000). Guidelines for end-of-life care in nursing homes: Principles and recommendations. Available at: www.hartfordign.org/policy/positions/guidelines_end_of_life.html.

Miller, S.C. (2003). Improving care in nursing homes-The integration of palliative care. Power Point presentation available at: www.capc.org/site_root/Files/1

National Nursing Home Survey (1999). Available at www.cdc.gov/nchs/data/nnhsd/ NNHS599selectedchar_homes_beds_residents.pdf

Orloff-Kaplan, K., Urbina, J., & Koren, M. (2000). Moving palliative care upstream: Integrating curing and caring paradigms in long term care. Unpublished background paper. The Fan Fox and Leslie R. Samuels Foundation with Partnership for Caring.

Petrisek, A.C., & Mor, V. (1999). Hospice in nursing homes: A facility-level analysis of the distribution of hospice beneficiaries. *Gerontologist*, 39, 279-290.

Rosenthal-Masella, S., Sansone, P., & Phillips, M. (2004). Palliative care in nursing homes, steps for success: A guide to developing a quality palliative care program. Available at www.scherviercares.org/pc_booklet.pdf

Teno, J.M. (2002). Now is the time to embrace nursing homes as a place of care for dying persons. Innovations in End-of-Life Care. 4(2).

Teno, J.M., Weitzen, S., Wetle, T., & Mor, V. (2001). Persistent pain in nursing home patients. *Journal of the American Medical Association*, 285(16):788.

Tuch, H., Parrish, R., & Romer, A. L. (2002). Integrating palliative care into nursing homes: An interview with Howard Tuch and Pam Parish. Innovations in End-of-Life Care, 4(2). Available at: <http://www2.edc.org/lastacts/archives/archives March02/featureinn.asp>

United Hospital Fund (2001). Voices of decision in nursing homes: Respecting resident's preference for end-of-life care. NY: The Fund. [WT 27.1 U58 2001].

von Gunten, C., Ferris, F., & Emmanuel, D'Antuono (2002). Recommendations to improve end-of-life care through regulatory change in U.S. health care financing. *Journal of Palliative Medicine*, 5(1):35-41.

World Health Organization (2004). The solid facts, Palliative care, Available at www.euro.who.int/document/E82931.pdf

Zerzan, J., Stearns, S., & Hanson, L. (2000). Access to palliative care and hospice in nursing homes. *Journal of the American Medical Association*, 284(19):2489-2494.

3
Patient-Centered Palliative Care in the Home

Francine Rainone DO PhD MS* and Marlene McHugh MS RN FNP

1. Introduction

In America and other wealthy countries, the average life expectancy has increased and the burden of acute illness has decreased dramatically during the twentieth century (Covinsky *et al.*, 1994). Contemporary Americans overwhelmingly die from chronic, progressive diseases (Glaser and Strauss, 1968). In their last years, chronic disease(s) and increasing disability challenge the resources of most Americans. Changes in the family structure (including smaller size), increased likelihood that children live at some distance from their parents, and the fact that most families require that two people work in order to be financially viable, mean that family members are less likely than in prior generations to be able to provide the increased levels of care required by aging relatives (Lynn and Adamson, 2003). Data from the Study to Understand Prognosis and Preferences for Outcomes and Risk of Treatments (SUPPORT) study indicate that when family members do provide this care, it requires significant sacrifices: almost one third of families spend down to poverty in order to care for their dying loved ones (Lunney *et al.*, 2003). Despite the evident need for assistance, family members received inadequate information about existing community services to which they were entitled. Managing the current patterns of old age and death requires changes in the way health care is conceived, delivered and financed. Here we primarily focus on the role of Palliative Care in the changes in the *conception and delivery* of health services.

The emerging discipline of Palliative Care represents a new conceptual approach to illness. Rather than being based on tissue and organ systems (e.g., cardiology and hematology), disease type (e.g., infectious disease, oncology)

FRANCINE RAINONE ● Medical Director, Palliative Care, Abington Memorial Hospital, 1200 Old York Road, Abington, PA 19001-3788. MARLENE McHUGH ● Associate Director, Palliative Care, Montefiore Medical Center, 111th East 210th Street, Bronx, New York 10467 and *Corresponding author: Medical Director, Palliative Care, Abington Memorial Hospital, 1200 Old York Road, Abington, PA 19001-3788.

or on age (e.g., pediatrics, adult medicine), Palliative Care takes what might be called a developmental approach to medical conditions. As people reach a certain stage in the development of their illnesses, the trajectory of their lives enters the palliative phase. Consequently, palliative care may be appropriate for people of all ages and most diseases. Data from the Bronx Community Palliative Care Initiative indicate that approximately 2% of patients attending community health centers fit into this category (Rainone *et al.*, 2007).

Building on work by Glaser and Strauss (1968), Lunney *et al.*, (2003) divided chronic disease into three types: nonfatal chronic illness, serious and eventually fatal chronic illness, and frailty. They identify three trajectories for the course of chronic disease. The first trajectory involves a short period of evident decline, typical of cancer. The second trajectory is characteristic of organ system failure, and involves long-term limitations with intermittent periods of exacerbation and partial recovery, and eventual death during an exacerbation. The third trajectory involves prolonged dwindling, and is typical of dementia, disabling stroke and frailty. Regardless of trajectory, Palliative Care may be conceived as addressing the comprehensive health needs of people with *progressive functional decline, whose life will be limited by disease but whose remaining life span is unpredictable*. They constitute a service group not because of age or diagnosis but because they suffer from increasing numbers, severity and duration of their illnesses and disabilities.

However advanced its conceptualization of disease trajectory, Palliative Care emerged within a system of health care delivery organized by settings – outpatient clinics, hospitals, homes, and institutions providing long term care. The current system of reimbursement is primarily oriented to delivering health care in hospitals and clinics, and financially privileges interventional procedures over the kind of labor-intensive care typically needed by people with increasing frailty and disability. In this chapter we argue for four premises: 1) that providing services in the home is essential to adequate Palliative Care; 2) that the philosophy of Palliative Care entails a patient-centered approach rather than a setting/disease-centered approach to service delivery; and 3) that primary care providers are better positioned to provide patient-centered home palliative care than hospital-based specialists. Finally, we argue 4) that primary care providers need to form partnerships with nursing and community service organizations to provide continuity based home palliative care services.

2A. The Home is an Essential Setting for Palliative Care

Currently the bulk of Palliative Care services are delivered in the hospital. In that setting the focus is limited in scope: acute symptom management of advanced incurable disease, resolution of conflict over goals of care, formalization of advance directives, withdrawal of life prolonging therapies and assistance with referral to home care and hospice services. Outpatient palliative care clinics providing follow up to acute care constitute a second setting. In addition to follow up, these outpatient clinics handle the bulk of chronic pain patients. Increasingly, attempts are being made to use outpatient clinics as settings for providing palliative care early in the course of a disease. For example, cancer patients experiencing side effects to treatment may be seen by Palliative Care specialists rather than being managed exclusively by their oncologists or surgeons.

From the patient's perspective, it may be impractical or impossible to access outpatient palliative care clinic resources. To begin with, for a patient who must follow up with an oncologist, a radiation oncologist and a surgeon, an additional visit to an additional provider may neither be welcome nor result in improved care. For patients with multiple disabilities and/or symptoms, transportation to medical appointments is often limited by reliance on caregivers who themselves have multiple responsibilities. When family members have exhausted their family medical leave benefits, symptoms arise suddenly, or transportation is only available during evening and weekend hours when clinics are usually closed, the Emergency Department may appear to be the most convenient source of medical care. However, most Emergency Departments are not prepared to manage palliative care patients; costly and repetitive or unnecessary tests and treatments may be pursued, and non-emergent utilization of these services places further burdens on this congested setting.

To date there is no consensus on whether, when or how Palliative Care services should be provided at home, except within the context of Hospice. The Medicare Hospice benefit is intended for people with a life expectancy of six months or less, who forego curative treatment. Where life expectancy is uncertain, Hospice may not be appropriate. Expanding on their earlier work, Lunney *et al.* (2003) identified five patterns of *functional decline to death*. These are: sudden death, death from cancer, death from organ failure, death from frailty, and a fifth group characterized by modest and gradual decline in functional status (those with ischemic heart disease constituted the largest proportion of this group). People on different trajectories have different medical needs. Those who die suddenly bring home forcefully the need for each of us to complete advance directives, but obviously do not need home palliative care. Compared to decedents from sudden death, decedents from frailty are 8 times more likely to be dependent in activities of daily living (ADLs), decedents from cancer 1.5 times more likely, and decedents from organ failure 3 times more likely. Cancer decedents are relatively more dependent in ADLs in the last 3 months of life. The current Medicare Hospice benefit is most suitable for people with conditions like cancer, because its final stages follow a generally predictable course (Noelker, 2001), facilitating identification of Hospice eligibility. In contrast, prognosis for frail decedents is less reliable, and they are relatively more dependent the entire last year of their lives. For those with organ failure, decline in function is erratic, and prognosis is uncertain even in the last days of life (Lynn *et al.*, 1997). The uncertainty around prognostication partly accounts for the continued underutilization of home hospice care for patients at the end of life. In 2003 only 38% of patients with anticipated death were receiving home hospice care and in 2002 the national median duration of hospice care was only three weeks (Hastings Center, 2003).

Those who die from progressive frailty and organ failure constitute the group most likely to benefit from ongoing Palliative Care at home in the last years of their life. Data from Medicare claims indicate that three-fifths of Americans follow one of these patterns of decline to death (Lunney *et al.*, 2002). Currently, Palliative Care specialists see these patients in the hospital during times of acute crisis, with virtually no follow up by the specialist if the patient is discharged. Most hospital based palliative care teams are small, comprised of a social worker, advance practice nurse, physician and possibly a pastoral care provider. Preliminary data indicate that such teams can effectively provide service to about 40 new hospital-based patients per month and at best can conduct only sporadic home visits (O'Mahony *et al.*, 2005). If we agree that the patient's palliative care needs do not end at the hospital door, the limitations of this system are apparent.

2B. Current System of Home Care

In 2002, more than one million patients in the United States were receiving skilled homecare services, and many of them had significantly advanced chronic illnesses (National Center for Health Statistics, 2002). Medicare is the major funder for these services. There are three criteria for eligibility: the person must have Medicare Part A or Part B coverage under the original plan or be in a managed Medicare plan; s/he, must meet Medicare criteria for being homebound; and s/he must need *skilled* care by a nurse, physical therapist occupational therapist or speech therapist on an *intermittent* [fewer than 7 days per week, or less than 8 hours per day for 21 days or less www.ssa.gov] basis. S/he must also be unable to leave home without considerable and taxing effort [http://www.medicare.gov/Pulications/Pubs]. The skilled nursing services currently covered by this benefit are in four categories: observation and assessment; teaching and training; skilled treatments and procedures; and management and evaluation of a care plan. Observation and assessment is indicated when there is a risk of complications or repeated acute illness. Teaching and training involves explaining tasks that the patient or caregivers will then assume themselves. Skilled treatments and procedures are paid for unless/until the patient/ caregiver can assume the. Management and evaluation of a care plan is covered when necessary for the safety or recovery of the patient.

At present, home care is dominated by nursing services. Community based organizations such as the Visiting Nurse Service of New York (VNSNY) have established centers of excellence that utilize evidence based protocols to deliver home care for a wide variety of chronic illnesses and conditions, ranging from wound care to stroke, heart failure and chronic obstructive pulmonary disease. The availability of intravenous medications, wound and ostomy care, and portable imaging that can be transmitted over phone lines has revolutionized home care. Utilizing Information Technology to link nurses in the field with supervisors, these home programs allow for centralized record keeping and fast responses to patients' needs. Many large hospitals have home care teams managed by nurses that follow patients on discharge. On a smaller scale, physician home visits also have increased. The American Academy of Home Care Physicians is a growing organization that offers a Home Care Credentialing Exam. A growing number of community organizations and hospitals operate teams of home care physicians who bring primary care to those unable to travel to medical appointments.

Unfortunately, the growth in service provision apparently has not resulted in improved care. Family members of patients receiving homecare at the end of life rate the service as excellent in only 50% of cases when care is provided by non-Hospice organizations and only 70% of cases when provided by Hospice (Teno *et al.*, 2004). And notably, whether nurses or physicians deliver home care, it is rare that the same team follows a patient from home through hospitalization and back.

3. Promises to Keep: A Patient-Centered Approach to Delivering Palliative Care

Lynn and Adamson (2003) articulate seven promises integral to any reliable system of care for the chronically ill at the end of their lives. Four of these promises concern the delivery of care: no gaps in care, no surprises in the course of care, customized care and consideration for family situations. Although they do not use the terminology, the seven promises delineate the essential aspects of what primary care providers and others call *patient-centered care*.

Patient-centered care is based on a partnership among health care providers, patients and (when appropriate) the patients' families (Mead and Bower, 2000). In accordance with this philosophy, delivery of services is organized so that the preferences and values of individuals are respected, to the maximal degree possible. The Institute of Medicine (IOM) 1997 report on End-Of-Life care emphasized the principle of continuity of care, and this principle has been endorsed by a diverse range of medical specialties and professional organizations (Field and Cassel, 1997). In later reports the IOM expanded on this concept, and it now regards patient-centered care as essential to improving the quality of health care systems (Swift and Corrigan, 2000).

Customizing care to individual preferences and responding to family values and needs is already an essential part of Palliative Care. However, when it comes to eliminating gaps in care the current delivery of Palliative Care is part of the problem, not the solution. Gaps in care are disruptions in continuity. Several kinds of disruption affect patient care. The four major types are disruption of services, setting, medical information and providers.

3.1. Gaps in Services and Settings

Disruption of services is often linked to a change in settings. Each move among the settings of home, hospital, rehabilitation facility and nursing home requires arranging for multiple services to follow the patient. Providing continuity of services may require navigating the requirements of multiple agencies. Social workers have become skilled at ensuring that essential services remain in place across settings. However, the need to coordinate with multiple agencies, many of which are unable to initiate service on weekends and holidays, often delays discharge from the hospital, which exposes patients to risk of infection and needlessly adds to the cost of care.

3.2. Gaps in Medical Information

Disruptions in the flow of medical information occur when important information does not travel with the patient from provider to provider and/or setting to setting. Numerous efforts to expand and adapt information technology to ensure provision of accurate, portable, complete medical information are underway (Kibbe *et al.*, 2004). At present, however, Living Wills, Do Not Resuscitate orders and Health Care Proxies, even when they exist, are often missing from the medical chart when a patient transfers to another setting. Their absence may lead to unwanted or unnecessary interventions. Discontinuities in medical information are magnified by multiple delivery systems and organizations with limited mechanisms for communication across organizations.

3.3. Gaps in Continuity

The gap in Palliative Care that has received the least attention is lack of continuity of providers. Two reviews of provider continuity in primary care reached similar conclusions: multiple studies indicate that continuity of providers is associated with increased preventive services, decreased hospitalizations and emergency department visits (Cabana and Jee, 2004) and increased patient satisfaction (Cabana and Jee, 2004: Saultz and Albedaiwi, 2004). None of the reviewed studies addressed Palliative Care specifically, but several of them concerned patients with chronic disease, who would be considered eligible for home Palliative Care.

These studies of the value of continuity in care cannot be directly compared with the studies that show decreased hospitalizations and increased satisfaction from home care services that do not provide continuity. As a result, the evidence does not indicate the relative weight of the many variables at issue.

What is clear is that when the same providers follow a patient across settings, there is no gap in information and a decreased risk of gaps in services.

4. Palliative Care at Home: The Case for Primary Care

The first principle of palliative care is non-abandonment. This principle is expressed within many specialty areas of medicine. The foundations of family medicine in particular are congruent with the goals of the emerging discipline of Palliative Care. The five principles of family medicine are: access to care; continuity of care; comprehensive care; coordination of care; and contextual care. These principles overlap with those governing palliative care. In addition, the centrality of the physician-patient relationship in family medicine places the principle of non-abandonment at the heart of the discipline.

Family medicine, like Palliative Care, is and has always been intrinsically patient-centered, team-oriented, and sensitive to the needs of the individual in the context of the family and community. The definition and philosophy of family medicine are articulated on the web site of the American Academy of Family Physicians (www.aafp.org):

"Family practice is a three-dimensional specialty, incorporating . . . (1) knowledge, (2) skill, and (3) process. While knowledge and skill may be shared with other specialties, the family practice process is unique. At the center of this process is the patient-physician relationship with the patient viewed in the context of the family. It is the extent to which this relationship is valued, developed, nurtured and maintained that distinguishes family practice from all other specialties.

. . .The family physician's care utilizes knowledge of the patient in the context of the family and the community. . . refers the patient when indicated to other sources of care while preserving continuity of care. The family physician's role as a cost-effective coordinator of the patient's health services is integral to the care provided. If the patient is hospitalized, this role prevents fragmentation and a lack of coordination of care."

As currently structured, Palliative Care lacks this emphasis on continuity.

The Program of All-inclusive Care for the Elderly (PACE) comes closest to utilizing the family medicine model of delivering health services for patients nearing the end of life (Reuben *et al.*, 1997). PACE provides comprehensive care by a multidisciplinary team. Based on the British day hospital, it integrates acute and long-term care. In return for monthly capitation payments from Medicare and Medicaid, programs assume full financial risk for the care of its patients and provide comprehensive care, including skilled nursing care, caregiver support, medical and social work visits, physical and occupational therapy, prescription medications, durable medical equipment and sometimes bereavement services and pastoral care. Service utilization is not capitated and cost shifting is avoided. Those who are not dually eligible (for Medicare and Medicaid) can pay out of pocket for services not covered by Medicare.

Since its beginnings in the 1970s, PACE has expanded to include 73 programs in 18 states. (www.npaonline.org, 2005). People who are at least 55 years old, are certified by their home state as eligible for nursing home care and live in the program's catchment area may enroll in PACE. Its goal is to maximize independence and reduce preventable hospitalizations and long-term institutionalizations through the provision of interdisciplinary homecare. PACE programs have had significant impact on short-term hospitalization and only 8% of PACE deaths occur in acute care hospitals (Weiland *et al.*, 2000).

PACE programs organize care delivery around day health centers. Patients are brought to the center, usually three days a week, where they are given meals, participate in a variety of activities, and also have appointments with the members of the team. Attendance at the center is individualized, and ranges from once a month to several times a week. Transportation to all appointments is included in the program. Because multiple providers closely observe patients, changes in status can be identified early, and appropriate interventions made to prevent further decline. In addition, each case is reviewed quarterly, and adjustments to the plan are discussed at the team level. PACE programs close the gaps in services, settings, information and continuity. The same team follows patients across all settings. If a patient requires hospitalization, his/her primary care provider is the attending of record. Should a patient require care in a skilled nursing facility, the PACE program would cover the costs and the same team would oversee the management. Frequent review also provides the opportunity for ongoing discussion about advance directives, goals and preferences for care.

While it would be difficult to demonstrate quantitatively, it is *prima facie* likely that because discussions of goals of care are routinely held with patients and families are educated about what to expect, there is a lower rate of utilizing/requesting medically futile interventions among those who participate in PACE programs. One of the barriers to withdrawing unnecessary and burdensome interventions on patients seen by the authors' hospital consult service is that the Palliative Care team is often the first to address prognosis with patients and their families. We hypothesize that holding these conversations earlier in the course of the disease would substantially reduce the frequency with which patients and their families experience conflict over decisions regarding limiting treatments that are unlikely to prolong life.

PACE programs use primary care practitioners – usually geriatricians - for chronic disease management and Palliative Care. While the PACE programs were targeted to the frail elderly, their applicability to patients with organ failure is obvious. Conversations about collaboration between PACE and Hospice are ongoing (Ryan *et al.*, 2004). The barriers are not due to philosophy so much as to the intricacies of the ways in which provision of health care is currently reimbursed. In 1998 PACE programs were allowed to apply for permanent provider status under Medicare. Those who enroll in PACE give up their Medicare benefits, including Hospice. Future collaborations will have to overcome regulatory barriers in order be accessible to the largest number of people.

Analogously, decisions about whether Primary Care Providers or hospital-based specialists should provide Palliative Care at home have more to do with regulations and systems of reimbursement than about patient-centered care.

The PACE model is an important alternative to Hospice, but it is unlikely to fill the entire spectrum of needs for Palliative Care in the community. Many patients with frailty, and even more patients with organ failure, particularly those with COPD and/or Heart Failure, are not eligible for nursing homes, and therefore are not eligible for PACE, but would benefit from a palliative approach. A different kind of partnership will be required for many of these individuals.

5. Partnerships for Improved Palliative Care

5.1. The Role of Nursing

The nursing profession has deep historical roots in care of the patient and family in the home setting. In the 1890's two young nurses, Lillian Wald and Florence Brewster, realized the need to provide care to impoverished immigrants newly relocated from Europe to the Lower East-Side of New York. Their vision helped define the role of public health and community based nursing care in America. The initial home care nursing agency was called the Henry Street Visiting Nurse Service, later known as the Visiting Nurse Service of New York (VNSNY). (www.vnsny.org, 2006).

In many organizations like VNSNY it is now common for registered nurses to provide home care to patients with multiple chronic disease processes. Such management requires expertise in high tech medical equipment, complex pharmacologic regimes, wound care and advanced physical assessment skills. The home care registered nurse is also the care coordinator for the patient and family in the community. As care coordinator, the home care nurse assesses the needs of the patient and family for psychosocial interventions, physical therapy, occupational therapy and various other professional interventions, and suggests appropriate consultation to the patient's primary care provider.

As a result of the increased complexity of care needs of patients and families, home care agencies have begun to incorporate Nurse Practitioners into the home care agency. The role of the advanced practice nurse varies, but in the VNSNY model, "the nurse practitioner provides education to the staff nurse around complex care needs and provides primary care management to patients as needed." (Mitty and Mezey, 1998). To date, community-based nursing organizations have not incorporated physicians into their supervisory structures.

5.2. Physician/Nurse Practitioner Teams

In contrast, community physicians sometimes partner with nurse practitioners to provide home care as a team. A nurse practitioner works in collaboration with a physician providing primary care to deliver services, including palliative care, to patients and families in the home setting. The nurse practitioner brings expertise in primary and chronic care management, technology, community health, quality improvement activities and case management to the home-bound patient. The physician brings medical expertise and decision-making skills in managing complex medical and psychiatric processes across treatment settings. Both providers are reimbursed for the primary health care services they provide in the home setting. Medicare reimburses nurse practitioners at 85% of the physician home visit fee (Cestari and Currier, 2001).

5.3. *Hospices, Physicians and Home Health Agencies*

Hospices can contract with home care agencies to provide specific time limited services. The services are paid within the existing Certified Home Health Agency (CHHA) reimbursement system. For home health agencies, reimbursement is under the Prospective Payment System based on the patient's Home Health Resource Group. The service must be provided for an indication other than that for which the patient is eligible for CHHA service (Raffa, 2003). The provision of palliative homecare is time intensive and requires specific expertise and training. By partnering with a hospice organization, CHHAs which do not have trained staff may benefit financially (Hanley, 2004). Hospice physicians can conduct a one time palliative care consultation in the home for patients receiving care from a CHHA, providing counseling of patients and families on end-of-life issues, care options and advance directives as well as a focus on pain and symptom management. Since the physician receives payment through Medicare Part B for these services, there is no increment in expenditure for the homecare organization (Hanley, 2004).

Some hospitals have begun programs with services targeted to homebound, chronically ill patients who do not have primary care providers. Such patients are very likely to lack preventive services and use the Emergency Department as their primary source of care. Developing a system that provides them with care by physicians or nurse practitioners who follow up with these patients at home improves continuity and could decrease burdensome, inappropriate visits to the Emergency Department. Unfortunately, in many of these programs, home care physicians and nurse practitioners do not follow their patients when they are admitted to hospital. In addition, until now their activities have not been coordinated with Palliative Care specialists, and there is no indication that they are required to maintain proficiency in Palliative Care.

All of these contractual arrangements among agencies multiply the number of providers tending to any particular patient, potentially fragmenting their care even further. We hypothesize that the multiplicity of agencies and providers partially explains why only 50% of family members of patients receiving homecare at the end-of-life rate the services as excellent (Teno *et al.*, 2004). This fragmentation is unlikely to be overcome without substantial changes to the way in which services are delivered and reimbursed.

Some Palliative Care specialists make a limited number of home visits as follow up to hospital care. There is no agreement on who should receive such visits, and multiple barriers exist to their routinization. Home visits are time intensive, and involve labor-intensive billing requirements. Reimbursement currently does not match the levels of energy required to integrate home care into routine palliative care.

6. Reflections on the Future of Palliative Home Care

Hospital-based Palliative Care has demonstrated that a multidisciplinary team involving, physicians, nurses, social workers and chaplains, which includes other disciplines as needed, provides the highest, most comprehensive level of care. We suggest that palliative home care requires the same mix of disciplines. At present, creating these teams may require partnerships among multiple organizations. However, "outsourcing" Palliative Care tasks is unlikely to be a long-term solution for any agency that wishes to maintain high standards.

Palliative Care is caught within the contradictions of the system it hoped to reform. Espousing an ideal of total care of the patient in the context of family and community, it is one more specialty in a system that is increasingly fragmented into ever more specialties, each one with increasingly narrower sets of responsibilities. The discontinuities of contemporary life, in which people rarely live their whole lives in the same region and rarely live in close proximity to the same friends for decades at a time, are mirrored in the lack of relationships with the same physician over the major portion of one's life.

In order to create an effective partnership among patients, families and providers several deficiencies need to be addressed. All providers need training in entitlements and community resources. Without knowing what services patients are able to receive, plans of care are often unrealistic. Given the complexity of illness and co-morbid conditions, primary care providers also need an educational curriculum which emphasizes geriatric pharmacology, polypharmacy, critical care management, and management of technology in the community. They will need to be familiar with new and emerging medical technologies. The Education for Physicians on End of Life Care (EPEC) project of the American Medical Association provides a comprehensive curriculum for physicians that address many of these needs. The End of Life Nursing Education Consortium (ELNEC), sponsored by the American Association of the College of Nursing and Nurse Researchers, serves a similar function for nurses (Emanuel et al., 1999; Paice et al., 2006; Matzo et al., 2003; Sherman et al., 2002). Both employ train-the-trainer curricula and two and a half day intensive courses. At local levels, a number of medical and nursing schools offer intensive courses in palliative care, of varying lengths, for health care providers.

Continuity of care also means that help is available 24 hours a day and seven days a week, requires knowledge of technology in the home setting and how to assess and manage situations when they arise in the home. This kind of coverage is already provided by many home care nursing agencies and managed care companies through nurse call centers.

Although the hospital was the right place for its birth, Palliative Care will not mature into the patient-centered, comprehensive service it espouses without expanding into community health centers. We also suggest that primary care providers should provide leadership in developing multidisciplinary teams that provide palliative home care. Maintaining the role of the primary care practitioner as care coordinator would establish continuity of care while still allowing for specialty consultation when needed. Patients' families could continue to receive care from their primary practitioners after the patients' deaths. Partnering home care nursing agencies with primary care practitioners would ensure that gaps in care were minimized, and respect for patients' values was maximized. There is a growing literature on ethnic and cultural variations in preferences for end of life care (Braun et al., 2000). It is clear that delivery of services will need to be modified in light of these differences. Rooted in the communities they serve, providers at health centers are well positioned to make these modifications.

As a subspecialty, Palliative Care is following the same course as Geriatrics. While some geriatricians are more hospital-based than others, in order to provide continuity of care it is the provider that follows patients across settings. Most geriatricians balance their time between the outpatient and inpatient settings, with the majority of time spent in the outpatient setting. Palliative and primary care providers who do not want to abandon their patients during their final passage would do well to follow their example.

References

Braun K, Pietsch J, Blanchette P, Eds. Cultural Issues in End-of-Life Decision Making. Sage Publications, Thousand Oaks, CA, 2000.

Cabana MD, Jee SH. Does continuity of care improve patient outcomes? J of Fam Prac 2004; 53(12):974-980.

Cestari L. and Currier, E. (2001). Caring for the Homebound Elderly: A Partnership between Nurse Practitioners and Primary Care Physicians. Home Health Care Management and Practice, Volume 13 #5 pp. 356-360.

Covinsky KE, Goldman L, Cook EF, et al. The impact of serious illness on patients' families. JAMA 1994; 272:1839-1844.

Emanuel LL, von Gunten CF, Ferris FD eds. The education for physicians on End-of-life care (EPEC) curriculum. EPEC Project. The Robert Wood Johnson Foundation, 1999.

Field MJ, Cassel CK eds. Washington DC:National Academic Press. Institute of Medicine (IOM) 1997. Approaching death: improving care at the End of Life, Institute of Medicine.

Glaser B, Strauus AL. Time for dying. Chicago, IL:Aldine Publishing Co:1968.

Hastings Center, National Hospice Work Group 2003, NHPCO 2004.

Hanley E. The role of homecare in palliative care services. Care Management Journals 2004; 5(3):151-157.

Institute of Medicine. Crossing the quality chasm: a new health system for the 21st century. National Academy Press, Washington, D.C., 2001.

Kibbe DC, Phillips RL, Green LA. The continuity of care record. Editorial. Am Fam Phys 2004; 70(7):1219.

Lynn J, Adamson DM, Rand White Paper. Living well at the end of life. Adapting health care to serious chronic illness in old age. 2003, p. 4.

Lynn J, Harell Jr. F, Cohn F, et al. Prognoses of seriously ill hospitalized patients on the days before death: implications for patient care and public policy. New Horiz 1997; 5(1):56-61.

Lunney JR, Lynn J, Foley DJ, Lipson S, Guralnik, J. Patterns of functional decline at the end of life. JAMA 289(18):2387-2392, 2003.

Lunney JR, Lynn J, Hogan C. Profiles of Older Medicare Decedents. J Am Geriatr Soc 2002; 50(6):1108-1122.

Matzo ML, Sherman DW, Penn B, Ferrell BR. The end-of-life nursing education consortium (ELNEC) experience. Nurse Educator. 28(6):266-70, Nov-Dec 2003.

Mead N, Bower P. Patient-centeredness: a conceptual framework and review of the empirical literature. Social Science and Medicine Oct 2000; 51(7):1087-1110.

Mitty, E. and Mezey, M. (1998). Integrating Advanced Practice Nurses in Home Care: Recommendations for a Teaching Home Care Program. Nursing and Health Care Perspectives, Volume 19(9) pp. 264-270.

National Center for Health Statistics 2004. National home and hospice care survey February 2004. http://www.cdc.gov/nchs/data/nhhcsd/curhomecare.pdf

National PACE Association website, www.npaonline.org, accessed 11/17/05.

Noelker, L. The backbone of the long-term-care workforce. Generations, 25(1); 2001.

O'Mahony S, Blank A, Zallman L, Selwyn PA. The Benefits of a Hospital Based Inpatient Palliative Care Consultation Service: Preliminary Outcome Data. Journal of Palliative Medicine. 8(5):1033-1039, October 2005, pp. 85.

Paice JA, Ferrell BR, Virani R, Grant M, Malloy P, Rhome A. Appraisal of the Graduate End-of-Life Nursing Education Consortium Training Program. J Palliative Med. 9(2):353-360, Apr 2006.

Raffa CA. Palliative Care: The legal and regulatory requirements. Caring Magazine 2004:6-9

Rainone F, Blank AE, Selwyn PS. The early identification of palliative care patients: preliminary processes and estimates from urban, family medicine practices. American Journal of hospice and palliative medicine 24:2, 1-4:April/May 2007.

Reuben DB, Eng C, Pedulla J, Eleazer GP, McCann R, Fox N. Program of All inclusive Care for the elderly (PACE): an innovative model of integrated geriatric care and financing. JAGS 45(2):223-232, 1997.

Ryan S, Tuuk M, Lee, M. PACE and hospice: two models of palliative care on the verge of collaboration. Clinic in geriatric medicine 2004; 20(4):783-794.

Saultz JW, Albedaiwi W. Interpersonal continuity of care and patient satisfaction: a critical review. Annals of Fam Med. 2(5):445-451, Sept-Oct 2004. For a related discussion, see McWhinney IR. Fourth Annual Nicholas J. Pisacano Lecture: The Doctor, the Patient, and the Home: Returning to Our Roots. JABFP 1997; 10(6):430-435.

Sherman DW, Matzo ML, Rogers S, McLaughlin M, Virani R. Achieving quality care at the end of life: a focus of the End-of-Life Nursing Education Consortium (ELNEC) curriculum. J Prof Nursing. 18(5):255-262, Sept-Oct 2002.

Swift E, & Corrigan JM (Eds) Institute of Medicine (IOM). Committee on the National Quality Report on Health Care Delivery, Board on Health Care Services.

Envisioning the National Health Care Quality Report. National Academy Press: Institute of Medicine. 2000.

Teno J, Claridge BR, Casey V, Welch LC, Wetle T, Shield R, et al. Family Perspectives on end-of-life care at the last place of care. Journal of the American Medical Association 2004; 291(1):88-93.

Weiland D, Lamb VL, Sutton SR, Boland R, Clark M, Friedman S, Brummel-Smith K, Eleazer GP Hopsitalization in the program of all-inclusive care for the elderly (PAC): rates, concomitants, and predictors. Journal of the American Geriatric Society 2000; 48(11):1373-1380.

4
Hospice Care

Carolyn Cassin MPA

1. Introduction

1.1. End of Life Issues and the Need for Hospice

A crisis is looming in the American health care system. The population of the United States is ageing. Over the next quarter century, the number of people older than 85 years will double. The massive generation of baby boomers is moving rapidly toward old age, and the reality that 65 million Americans will grow old and face the end of life together over the next thirty years is cause for national alarm. At the heart of the crisis is not only, the fear that the cost of caring for these Americans may bankrupt an already fragile health care system, but also the fear that the kind of care provided at the end of life for all patients, regardless of age, is wholly inadequate and ineffective in meeting end of life health care needs. Over the past twenty-five years a little known program – hospice – has revolutionized at least one part of the health care system – end of life care. Hospice has become the health care system's safety net for the last phase of life. Unfortunately, it is also the most under-utilized benefit in the American health care system.

Hospice is a program of care for persons, in the last phases of an incurable disease, and their families or caregivers. Hospices provide palliative care, as opposed to curative care. The goal of hospice is to manage the physical, psychological, spiritual, social, and practical issues that present as a result of the dying process and continue for the family in the year long bereavement period that follows death. Hospice is provided in both home and facility based settings by an interdisciplinary team of professionals - physicians, nurses, medical social workers, therapists, counselors and volunteers - who coordinate an individualized plan of care for each patient and family. Hospice reaffirms the right of every person and family to participate fully in the final stage of life.

CAROLYN CASSIN, MPA • President & Chief Executive Officer, Continuum Hospice Care, 1775 Broadway, New York, New York 10036.

1.2. The Wrong Care at the Wrong Time in the Wrong Setting

Over one-third of terminally ill patients have substantial care needs (Jennings, 2003). The evidence suggests that the last phase of life is often characterized by prolonged dying, accompanied by substantial emotional and financial expense and inadequate support for patients and families. An exhaustive examination of care at the end of life by the Hastings Center, in collaboration with the National Hospice Workgroup, revealed that for most Americans the health care experience in the last months of life is "deplorable and in need of full reconstitution" (The Last Acts Coalition, 2002). The report concludes that:

Too many Americans approach death without adequate medical, nursing, social and spiritual support. In the last stage of a long struggle with incurable, progressive diseases – such as cancer, heart or lung disease, AIDS, Alzheimer's, Parkinson's or Lou Gerhig's disease – their pain is untreated or inadequately controlled. Their depression or other mental health problems are not addressed. Many debilitating physical symptoms rob them of energy, dignity and sometimes the will to carry on. Family members who provide care are stressed, inadequately supported by professionals, and ultimately are often rendered ill themselves by the ordeal. Patients who wish to remain at home, in familiar surroundings, are often forced to spend their final days or weeks in a hospital or nursing home (Jennings et al., 2003).

Therefore, one may characterize the care at end of life, simply as the wrong care at the wrong time in the wrong setting.

The 1995 SUPPORT (Study to Understand Prognosis and Preferences for Outcomes and Risks of Treatment) study characterized dying as "painful, lonely and invasive" (The SUPPORT investigators, 1995). The researchers found that: (1) 50% of dying patients suffered severe pain; high hospital resource use and caregiver burden; (2) 20% of family members quit work to provide care and experienced financial devastation and (3) 30% to 40% of family members lost most of their savings while caring for a dying relative. The authors also reported lack of satisfaction of family members with the provision of information about community resources such as hospice. Another study to shed light on unmet needs at the end of life and the first study to examine the quality of end-of-life care on a national level was the 2004 study conducted by Dr. Joan M. Teno and her colleagues. The researchers interviewed bereaved family members to assess the end-of-life care that patients had received in home and institutional settings. The researchers found that:

- *One in four people who died did not receive enough pain medication and sometimes received none at all. Inadequate pain management was 1.6 times more likely in a nursing home setting than in a home setting with hospice;*
- *One in two patients did not receive enough emotional support, according to the respondents. This was 1.3 times more likely to be the case in an institution;*

- *One in four respondents expressed concern over physician communication and treatment decisions;*
- *Twenty-one percent complained that the dying person was not always treated with respect. Compared with a home setting, this was 2.6 times higher for patients who died in a nursing home setting and three times higher in a hospital setting;*
- *Fifteen percent of respondents said that they do not believe the health care providers had enough knowledge about the patient's medical history to provide the best care; and*
- *Respondents whose loved ones received spa hospice in a home setting were the most satisfied. More than 70% rated hospice care as excellent in comparison with 50% percent whose loved ones were in nursing homes or at home with home health services* (Teno et al., 2004).

Another factor that contributes to poor care near, or at the end of life is aggressive treatment, usually provided in hospitals. Although the likelihood that a person will die in the hospital has decreased to almost 40%, the likelihood of undergoing a procedure during the terminal hospitalization increased from 17.8% to 30.8%. One in five who died, underwent mechanical ventilation during their terminal admission. Fifty percent underwent placement of feeding tubes, 60% underwent endotracheal intubation and 75% underwent cardiopulmonary resuscitation (Barnatto, 2004).

Not only is end-of-life care, as it is currently provided, the wrong care, provided at the wrong time, it is also provided in the wrong setting. Townsend and colleagues, in a prospective study of a random sample of patients with cancer and a life expectancy of less than one year, found that 58% of patients stated a preference for dying at home during their initial interview. Fifty percent of those who would have preferred to die at home, but who died in a hospital, could have died at home if there had been more supportive care available (Townsend et al., 1990). Despite their preference, 75% of Americans die in health institutions rather than at home. There is a marked increase in the proportion of those who die at home, when hospice is available. For those patients who died with hospice care, 50% died at home, 23% died in a nursing home, 7% died in a hospice unit, 9% died in a hospital, 7% died in a freestanding inpatient facility operated entirely by a hospice and 4% died in a residential care setting (Teno et al., 2004; Townsend et al., 1990).

2. The History of Hospice

The modern hospice movement in the U.S. was influenced by the work of Elisabeth Kubler-Ross's in the 1960s, which demystified death and dying and opened a debate on care of the dying for health care professionals and the public. In her book, *On Death and Dying: What The Dying Have To Teach Doctors, Nurses, Clergy And Their Own Family* (Kubler-Ross, 1969) which was published in 1969, she recorded her observations of how people faced a terminal illness by listening to them at the bedside. As a result of her observations she identified the emotional phases of the terminally ill: denial, anger, bargaining, depression and acceptance (Hospice and Palliative Nurses Association, 2002). During the 1970s, hospice leaders began meeting regularly to formulate model standards for the development of hospice care. The creation of the National Hospice Organization in 1978 provided a national forum for discussion and education of hospice professionals and the development of hospice standards. Although hospices multiplied rapidly during the 1970's, they did not become institutionalized until 1982 when Congress added hospice care as a Medicare Benefit when it enacted the Tax Equity and Fiscal Responsibility Act (TEFRA). TEFRA defined how hospice would be paid for under the Medicare benefit (Hospice and Palliative Nurses Association, 2002). In 1997, the National Hospice Organization published, *A Pathway for Patients and Families Facing Terminal Illness,* (Ryndes, 1997) and the National Hospice and Palliative Care Organization published *Standards of Practice for Hospice* in 2002 which fostered the establishment of universal standards and practices for hospice agencies (National Hospice and Palliative Care Organization, 2002).

3. What is Hospice?

3.1. Fundamental Concepts

The National Hospice and Palliative Care Organization (NHPCO) describes hospice as:

A specialized form of multidisciplinary health care which is designed to provide palliative care, alleviate the physical, emotional, social and spiritual discomforts of an individual who is experiencing the last phase of life due to the existence of a life-limiting, progressive disease, to provide supportive care to the primary caregiver and the family of the hospice patient (Hospice and Palliative Nurses Association, 2002).

Typically, a family member serves as the primary caregiver and, when appropriate, helps make decisions for the terminally ill individual. Members of the hospice staff make regular visits to assess the patient and provide additional care or other services. Hospice staff are on-call 24 hours a day, seven days a week. Hospice care also extends to the patient's loved ones, helping them cope with the many problems associated with the end of a loved one's life. Therefore, the patient's plan of care includes the family caregiver. Services to family caregiver(s) include: (1) instructions on caring for the patient; (2) emotional support and respite; (3) assistance and companionship from trained volunteers and (4) bereavement support for up to 13 months after the death of their loved one. Hospice makes it possible for patients and caregivers to use this final stage of life for life review, closure, and personal development.

3.2. Hospice Statistics

The NHPCO compiles annual statistical data on hospice membership, legal status, organizational structure, certification and accreditation, provision and utilization of services, and patient demographics (National Hospice and Palliative Care Organization, 2003). For the year 2003, there were approximately 3,300 operational hospice programs, in U.S in all fifty states, Puerto Rico and Guam; serving 850,000 patients (Figures 4.1 & 4.2) and families annually (National Hospice and Palliative Care Organization, 2003).

3.2.1. Types of Programs

Characteristics of U.S. hospice programs for the year 2003 are reflected in the charts below:

As indicated above, the role of government in providing hospice services is quite limited, except for reimbursement through the Medicare hospice benefit.

3.2.2. Patient Demographics

The characteristics of the 850,000 patients served by hospice for the year 2003 are as follows (see Tables 4.2 & 4.3):

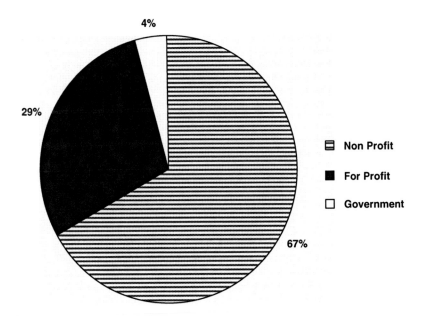

FIGURE 4.1.
Source: National Hospice and Palliative Organization, Facts and Figures. Research Department; 2003, www.nhpco.org, viewed on 12-1-04

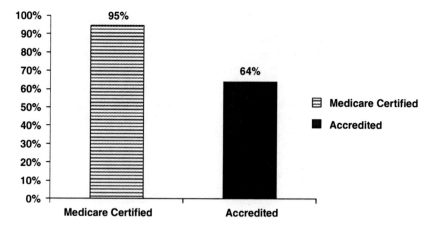

FIGURE 4.2.
Source: National Hospice and Palliative Care Organization, Facts and Figures, research
department; 2003, www.nhpco.org, viewed on 12-1-04

TABLE 4.1. Leading hospice diagnoses

Top hospice diagnosis	2003
Cancer	49.0%
End-stage heart disease	11.0%
Dementia	9.6%
COPD	6.8%
End stage kidney disease	2.8%
End stage liver disease	1.6%
Other	19.2%
Total	100%

Source: National Hospice and Palliative Care
Organization, Facts and Figures, research
department; 2003, www.nhpco.org, viewed on 12-1-04

Tremendous in-roads have been made in the last decade in the diversifica-
tion of the hospice patient base away from one that was disproportionately
cancer-based from 76 % in 1992 down to 49% in 2003 (Table 4.1). These trends
are likely to continue as more hospices reach out to patients who are dying
from illnesses other than cancer (General Accounting Office HEHS-00-182).

It should be noted that there are significant disparities in access to health
care between racial and ethnic groups and persons of different socioeconomic
status in the United States (Agency for Healthcare Research and Quality, 2000)
Race, ethnicity, and socioeconomic status are also correlated with differential
patterns in care received at the end of life. Hogan and colleagues recently inves-

TABLE 4.2. Sex of recipients of hospice care for 2003

Sex	Percentage
Male	54%
Female	46%

Source: National Hospice and Palliative Care
Organization, Facts and Figures, research
department; 2003, www.nhpco.org, viewed on 12-1-04

TABLE 4.3. Age of recipients of hospice care for 2003

Age	Percentage
Less than 75 years of age	37%
75 years of age or older	63%

Source: National Hospice and Palliative Care Organization,
Facts and Figures, research
department; 2003, www.nhpco.org, viewed on 12-1-04

TABLE 4.4. Race/Ethnicity of recipients of hospice care for 2003

Race/Ethnicity	Percentage
Caucasian or white (does not include hispanic or latino whites)	81.2%
Black or African-American	9.0%
Multicultural or another race	4.6%
Hispanic or Latino	4.3%
Asian or Hawaiian/Pacific Islander	0.9%

Source: National Hospice and Palliative Care Organization, Facts an Figures, research
department; 2003, www.nhpco.org, viewed on 12-1-04

tigated patterns in the use of care by Medicare beneficiaries in the 3 years
before death. They found that African Americans used 25% less care in the
3 years before death than Caucasians, but 18% more in the last year of life
(Table 4.4). The research above clearly indicates that there continues to be a
high level of unmet need within our healthcare system (Hogan *et al.*, 2001).

Median length of stay (LOS) is a more accurate way to understand the
experiences of typical hospice patients than average LOS (Figures 4.3 & 4.4).
The fact that over one-third of hospice patients died in seven days or less
reinforces that patients are not being referred to hospice in a timely manner.
This prevents them from reaping the full benefits of hospice. In 2003, 95.5%
of hospice care was provided as routine home care, 3.4% as general inpatient
care, 0.2% as respite care, and 0.9% as continuous care (National Hospice
and Palliative Care Organization, 2003).

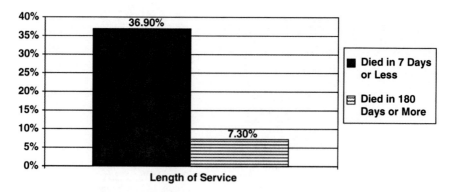

FIGURE 4.3. Length of Stay (LOS)
Source: National Hospice and Palliative Care Organization, Facts and Figures, research department; 2003, www.nhpco.org, viewed on 12-1-04

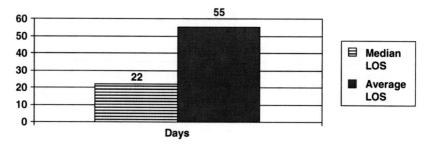

FIGURE 4.4. Median Length of Stay (MLOS)
Source: National Hospice and Palliative Care Organization, Facts and Figures, research department; 2003, www.nhpco.org, viewed on 12-1-04

3.3. The Role of Nursing Homes in Providing Hospice Care

In 2003, 25% of Americans died in nursing homes. For those patients who die under hospice care, 23% died in a nursing home. There are benefits to both the nursing home and the hospice. Hospices increase their revenue by adding to their patient census, more efficient utilization of staff and increased average length of stay on hospice. Nursing homes that enroll residents on hospice can increase their patient census by providing end-of-life care to individuals who can no longer remain at home and also reduce in-house staff time (hospice staff provide service to these patients) as well as adding specialized end-of-life services. A hospice may also agree to pay room and board rates that are equivalent to the rates that the nursing home would have received directly from government agencies. Hospice will also pay for durable medical equipment, prescriptions and other supplies related to the patient's terminal illness, which might not otherwise be reimbursed. A continued increase in the number of nursing home Medicare hospice beneficiaries therefore is likely. Although a 1999 study found that the number of nursing homes with hospice units doubled between 1992 and 1995 from 0.5% to 1.0%, less than 1% of residents per facility surveyed were identified as hospice beneficiaries on the day of the most recent inspection visit by the researchers (Petrisek, 1999).

3.3.1. Licensure and Accreditation

In 1998, 43 states licensed hospice organizations, using widely varying requirements. Hospices may also be licensed in other categories, usually as home health agencies or health facilities. In 1990, the Joint Commission incorporated requirements for hospice into its home care accreditation program. In 1992, however, standards for addressing the needs of dying patients were also developed and incorporated into the accreditation process for all health care settings. It should be noted that currently there is no mandatory nationwide certification or accreditation for hospice (Longest et al., 1998; Hospice and Palliative Nurses Association, 2002).

3.3.2. Staffing

Hospice organizations rely heavily on volunteers. In the year 2003, approximately 400,000 hospice volunteers contributed 10% of all hours of service provided by hospices. This is equal to over 18 million hours per year. (Hospice and Palliative Nurses Association, 2002). All Medicare hospice volunteers must participate in intensive volunteer training programs.

4. The Hospice Medicare/Medicaid Benefit

In the year 2003, 70% of hospice payments were through the Medicare program. In 2004, nearly 1,000,000 beneficiaries elected hospice care, according to the NHPCO. By 2004, almost every state had adopted a Medicaid hospice benefit and every major insurer has a hospice benefit included within its health insurance package (National Hospice and Palliative Care Organization, 2003).

4.1. Eligibility

Enactment of the Medicare hospice benefit requires (1) a physician to certify a medical prognosis of a life expectancy of six months or less, if the disease runs its normal course; (2) that the patient chooses to receive hospice care rather than curative treatments for their illness and (3) that the patient enrolls in a Medicare-approved hospice program. The Medicare Part A Hospice Benefit includes two 90 day periods, followed by unlimited subsequent periods of 60 days each. Both home health care and inpatient hospice are covered. The beneficiary must be recertified as terminally ill at the beginning of each benefit period by a physican (National Hospice and Palliative Care Organization, 2003; Longest, 1998).

4.2. Medicare Core Services

Under the Medicare hospice benefit the following core hospice services which are delienated in the Medicare Conditions of Participation, 42 CFR, 400-429, www.hospicepatients.org/law.html must be provided (see Table 4.5):

4.3. Interdisciplinary Team

Under the Medicare benefit the interdisciplinary team (IDT) plays a vital role in directing and coordinating care and ensuring that Medicare regulations are met. Coordination of care by the Team is vital as patients may move between different levels of care – routine home care, in-patient care, respite care or continuous care. The IDT includes the attending physician and hospice physicians, a registered nurse skilled in patient assessment and training in pain and symptom management, a social worker experienced in discharge planning and family counseling, spiritual counselors and bereavement counselors. Other team members may include occupational therapists, physical therapists, speech-language pathologists, music and art therapists, massage therapists, psychologists, and a wide range of community resource providers. All tests and treatments, drugs, durable medical equipment, and medical supplies identified by the team as necessary for the palliation of the terminal illness must also be provided to the patient (Longest, 1998).

4.4. The Role of the Physican

There are a number of benefits to a physician when recommending hospice to patients: (1) patients receive specialist level palliative care services at end of life; (2) the physician continues to manage the care of the patient; (3) the

TABLE 4.5. Medical core hospice services
- Nursing care
- Medical social worker
- Physician
- Dietary, pastoral and other counselors
- Home health aide and homemaker
- Short-term inpatient care including respite care and inpatient care for procedures necessary for pain control and acute and chronic system management
- Medical appliances and supplies, including drugs and biologicals; physical and occupational therapies; and speech-language pathology services
- Bereavement service for the family is provided for up to 13 months following the patient's death including educational programs about grief, group sessions, individual counseling, and routine contact from the hospice team

physician receives payment for care s/he provides either as an attending or as a consultant and (4) the physician becomes a member of the hospice IDT. Once admitted to hospice, the patient chooses an attending physician to become the "physician of record" who will work with the hospice to coordinate the patient's plan of care. This physician continues to be paid for any services delivered to the patient through the regular Part B payments s/he would normally receive. Payment for technical services (laboratory, x-rays, chemotherapy, radiation, etc.) must be billed to the hospice for payment and must be on the patient's plan of care before payment can be made. Other physicians can continue to be involved in the care of the hospice patient as consultants and receive reimbursement through the hospice program. These physicians must have a contract with the hospice and their services listed as necessary on the patient's hospice plan of care. (National Hospice and Palliative Care Organization *Providing Direct, Billable Physician Services to Hospice Patients: An Opportunity to Upgrade the Medical Component of Hospice Care*; www.nhpco.org).

4.5. Medicare Expenditures and Reimbursement

Medicare pays the hospice program a per diem rate that is intended to cover virtually all expenses related to addressing the patient's terminal illness. The Medicare Hospice Benefit affords patients four levels of care to meet their needs: (1) Routine Home Care (this category is for individuals receiving hospice care at home); (2) Continuous Home Care (individuals in this category must need skilled services for a period of at least eight hours within a 24-hour period beginning at midnight, but only for brief periods of crisis and only as necessary to maintain the terminally ill individual at home); (3) Inpatient Respite Care (may be provide for no more than five days at a time in an inpatient facility) and (4) General Inpatient Care may be provided in a Medicare-certified hospital, skilled nursing facility, or inpatient unit of a hospice (www.nhpco.org). Ninety-six percent of hospice care is provided at the routine home care level.

There have been a number of reports and studies that challenge the adequacy of the Medicare hospice benefit rates. One study, sponsored by the NHPCO and conducted by Millman USA, has come to this conclusion. The researchers analyzed data reported by Medicare certified hospice organizations and showed that the current Medicare reimbursement for routine home care does not cover the costs incurred by hospice organizations to deliver this service. For the 1998-1999 samples, they found that hospice costs exceed revenue by about 20%, and even assuming a much longer length of service, costs would still exceed revenue by 10% (Milliman, 2001). The researchers identified three factors that have contributed to hospice losses (1) the length of time patients actually receives hospice services - which has decreased resulting in an increase in per diem costs for each patient, while per diem income has remained flat; (2) the intensity of hospice services has increased dramatically

- which has resulted in an increase in the hospice cost per day and (3) the rapid growth in prescription drug and outpatient costs - which has contributed to an increase in hospice cost per day.

4.6. Cost Savings

There is evidence that hospice has proven to be a less costly approach to care for the terminally ill on both a national and state level. Much of the savings from hospice care relative to conventional care accrue in the last month of life, which is due, in large part, to the substitution of home care days for inpatient days during this period. In the last year of life, hospice patients receiving the Medicare benefit incurred approximately $2,737 less in cost than those not on the Medicare hospice benefit; saving totaled $3,192 in the last month of life (Lewin, 1995). In addition, in comparison to acute hospital and skilled nursing facility costs, hospice is a less costly service. For 1998, hospital inpatient charges per day were $2,177; skilled nursing facility charges per day were $482 and hospice charges per covered day of care were $113 (Health Care Financing Administration, 2000). More recently Bruce Pyenson and his colleagues sought to identify cost differences between patients who do and do not elect to receive Medicare-paid hospice benefits (Pyenson et al., 2004). This study provides evidence that, for certain well-defined terminally ill populations, costs are lower for patients who choose hospice care than for those who do not. Furthermore, for certain well-defined terminally ill populations, among the patients who died, patients who chose hospice care lived longer on average than similar patients who did not choose hospice care. The researchers found that this pattern persisted across most of the disease states studied. The researchers also found that hospice care was widely used by patients with cancer, which was reflected in the high proportion of patients choosing hospice care in their cancer diagnoses groups. Notable among the findings, however, is that the CHF – related group, where relatively few patients receive hospice care, showed lower cost and longer time until death for the patients who choose hospice care.

5. Problems Facing Hospice

5.1. Access and Misunderstanding

Although hospices currently serve nearly one out of every five deaths in the US, the option of hospice care is simply unknown to most patients and families and simply not known by most of America's physicians. Most startling is the lack of awareness, understanding or knowledge that health care professionals have about the hospice benefit. For example, few providers seem aware that hospice is an *entitlement* benefit – anyone with a Medicare, Medicaid card or private health care insurance has access to hospice, if they qualify for the services.

Why hasn't hospice become standard medical practice for every patient at end of life? Myths about hospice have contributed to its lack of full integration into the health care system.

Myth #1: This patient isn't hospice appropriate...they aren't close to dying, and they haven't given up hope

The difficulty over a physician's ability to prognosticate effectively the patient's six month life expectancy has plagued hospices since the requirement was crafted as an entry requirement to utilization of the Hospice Medicare benefit over twenty years ago. Several studies have demonstrated the difficulty physicians have in making certain the patient has only six months to live (Christakis, 1997; Christakis, 1998). Nicholas Christakis, MD, PhD has written extensively about how often physicians err in their prognosis in terminally ill patients. In 2000 he surveyed three hundred forty-three (343) physicians who provided survival estimates for 468 terminally ill patients at the time of hospice referral. His findings were:

- *Only 20% (92/468) of predictions were accurate (within 33% of actual survival); 63% (295/468) were overoptimistic and 17% (81/468) were over pessimistic*
- *Overall, doctors overestimated survival by a factor of 5.3*
- *As the duration of doctor-patient relationship increased and time since last contact decreased, prognostic accuracy decreased*

Dr. Christakis concluded that the inaccuracy is, in general, not restricted to certain kinds of doctors or patients and that these phenomena may be adversely affecting the quality of care given to patients near the end of life. With a median length of stay nationally at 22 days, there is little reason to believe that hospice patients are being referred too early. The benefit itself, is remarkably forgiving if prognosis has been incorrect and over estimated. Patients can revoke the benefit and return to regular Medicare if they choose to pursue curative rather than focus on palliative treatment. The early fear that physicians making an incorrect prognosis would somehow be penalized has not materialized. There have been no repercussions to physicians for late or even early referral to hospice.

Myth #2: The family and patient aren't ready to hear about hospice; they haven't acknowledged that the patient is dying

Fortunately, the requirements for hospice eligibility do not require that the patient in some way be "ready" to face death. In fact, most hospice programs would say that it is this particular expertise – that of helping the patient and family come to terms with the inevitability of death – which is the precise reason why terminally ill patients should be enrolled in a hospice program. To require patients and families to come to this realization prior to the hospice admission, denies them hospice's expertise in working through these difficult issues. Patients must acknowledge that they have a life limiting disease and that they understand that under the hospice program, they will not be pursuing treatment to cure the underlying cause of the disease. This conversation is usually off-putting for patients. In fact, nearly all patients readily acknowledge the life limiting nature of their illness and respond favorably to the help and services hospice has to offer.

Myth #3: Hospice isn't appropriate because the patient still wants "active" treatment for the disease, or "life sustaining" treatment

Nowhere in the philosophical underpinnings of hospice or the statutory or regulatory requirements that allow care to be provided is there a requirement that the patient must be willing to give up care to access hospice. Disease modifying therapies have always been permitted under the benefit although many hospices have refused to admit patients to their program until they had finished treatments, fearing both the financial burden to the hospice in addition to the need provide advanced clinical skills for patients undergoing active treatment.

6. Open Access – The Future of Hospice

With the full use of the hospice benefit for all eligible patients in the United States, the end of life experience for Americans will improve dramatically. Patients and families will experience better clinical, spiritual and social outcomes related to the last phase of life, and they will be more satisfied with the experience. Care of patients in the last phase of life will be far less costly. Increased access to specialist level palliative care through hospice will drive the development of a more sophisticated, appropriate and welcome set of services to all terminally ill patients. An innovative group of programs in the United States began meeting ten years ago as the National Hospice Work Group. Their goal was to advocate the full use of hospice for all patients at the end of life; they characterized this approach as "Open Access" hospice care. While all hospice programs that participate in the Medicare and Medicaid programs have a standardized set of services and conditions of participation they must adhere to and fulfill, there is wide discretion on the front end as to which patients a hospice will accept into its service. The Federal Government has allowed hospices to set their own admission criteria and exclude patients for virtually any reason, but most often it appears that screening occurs because the hospice program assesses that the patient's care may be costly or if the patient has any remaining ambivalence assesses that about the end of life experience.

Open Access Hospice constructs no such barriers to hospice admission. It restricts access to hospice to only two requirements, both of which are the statutory definitions for hospice care under the Medicare Hospice law:

- *The hospice must obtain a physician's certification that the patient has a prognosis of six months or less if the disease runs its expected course.*
- *The patient elects the Medicare Hospice benefit by consenting to care.*

The implications of reducing the eligibility requirements for hospice to these two factors are profound. Hospice patients may receive any treatment during their hospice experience unless it extends prognosis beyond six months. Hospice patients may continue to receive clinically and psychologically important treatments while still a hospice patient. Hospice patients can be referred earlier since there is no reason to wait until the patient completes treatment or is "ready to accept" hospice.

7. Conclusion

When hospice is properly utilized for the broad spectrum of patients in a community facing the last months of life, at least one aspect of the American health care system works effectively, efficiently and correctly. Patients and families get the care that they need and that they desperately want at the end of life. And most importantly, the American taxpayers benefit. Fewer dollars are spent on care and treatment that is not of the highest value to patients at the end of life. In the last months of life, patients and families value the opportunity to be pain free, comfortable and optimistic. They want the last months of life to be full and rewarding. They want to stay close to their family and friends, they want to be comforted by whatever religion or spiritual sense they rely on and most importantly, they want to understand how their life mattered to others. Hospice remains the only system that is designed and required to provide this full range of clinical, psychological and spiritual services.

References

Barnato, A., McClellan, M., Kagay, C., and Garber, A. (2004) Trends in inpatient treatment intensity among Medicare beneficiaries at the end of life – Practice patterns. *Health Services Research*. 39(2):363-75.

Christakis, N.A. and Iwashyna T.J. (1998) Attitude and self-reported practice regarding prognostication in a national sample of interns. *Arch Intern Med* 1998; 158 (21):2389-2395.

Christakis, N.A. (1999) *Death foretold: prophecy and prognosis in medical care.* Chicago, IL: University of Chicago Press.

Christakis, N.A. (1997) The ellipsis of prognosis in modern medical thought. *Soc Sci Med* 44:301-305.

Christakis, N.A. (2000) Extent and determinants of error in doctors': prognosis in terminally Ill patients: prospective cohort study. *BMJ.* 320(7233):469-472.

Field, M.J. and Cassel, C.K. (Eds.) (1997) Committee on Care at the End of Life, Division of Health Care Services. Institute of Medicine. *Approaching Death in America: Improving Care at the End of Life.* Washington: National Academy Press.

Hogan, C., Lynn, J., Gabel, J., Lunney, J., O'Mara, A., and Wilkinson, A. (2000) *Medicare beneficaries' costs and use of care in the last year of life.* Washington, DC. MedPAC. 00-1.

Hospice and Palliative Nurses Association, *Core Curriculum for the Generalist and Palliative Care Nurse,* 2002; Iowa: Kendall/Hunt Publishing Company.

Hospital and SNF Medicare Charge Data are from the *Annual Statistical Supplement, 2000,* to the *Social Security Bulletin,* Social Security Administration. The hospice charge data are from the *Health Care Financing Review, Statistical Supplement,* Health Care Financing Administration, 1997, 1998, 1999, and 2000.

Jennings, B., Ryndes, T., D'Onofrio, C., and Baily, M. (2003) *Hastings Center Report, Special Supplement, Access to Hospice Care: Expanding Boundaries, Overcoming Barriers* S2-S3.

Kubler-Ross, E. (1997) *On death and dying: what the dying have to teach doctors, nurses, clergy and their own family,* Scribner (re-print).

Lewin-VHI (1995). *An analysis of the cost Savings of the Medicare Hospice Benefit.* National Hospice Organization. Washington, DC.

Longest, B., Rakich, J., and Darr, K. (1998) *Managing health service organizations and systems,* "How health services organizations are organized" Illinois, Health Professions Press.

Miceli, P.J. and Mylod, D.E. (2003) Satisfaction of families utilizing end-of-life care: current successes and challenges within the hospice industry. *American Journal of Hospice and Palliative Care.* 20(5):360-370.

Miller, S.C., Mor, V., and Teno, J. (2003) Hospice enrollment and pain assessment and management in nursing homes. *J Pain Symptom Management* 26(3):791-799.

Millman USA *The cost of hospice care: an actuarial evaluation of the Medicare Hospice Benefit,* August 2001, found at www.nhpco.org/i4a/pages/index.cfm page 3368 (PDF file-TheCostofHospiceCare-millman.pdf), viewed on 1/20/05.

National Hospice and Palliative Organization, *Facts and Figures.* Research Department; 2003, found at www.nhpco.org, viewed on 12-1-04.

National Hospice and Palliative Care Organization, Hospice Facts and Statistics, found at www.nhpco.org/Consumer/hpcstats.html, viewed on 12-7-04.

National Hospice and Palliative Care Organization *Providing direct, billable physician services to hospice patients: an opportunity to upgrade the medical component of hospice care,* found at www.nhpco.org, viewed on 12-20-04.

National Hospice and Palliative Care Organization, *Standards of practice for hospice programs* (2002), found at www.nhpco.org, viewed on 1/24/05.

Petrisek, A. and Mor, V. (1999) Hospice in nursing homes: a facility-level analysis of the distribution of hospice beneficiaries. *Gerontologist* 39(3):279-90.

Pyenson, B., Connor, S., Fitch, K., and Kitzbrunner, B. (2004) Medicare cost in matched hospice and non-hospice cohorts. *J Pain Symptom Manage.* 28(3)200-10.

Ryndes, T. (1997) *A pathway for patients and families facing terminal illness.* Alexandria, VA: The National Hospice Organization.

SUPPORT Principal Investigators. (1995) A controlled trial to improve care for seriously ill hospitalized patients. The Study to Understand Prognoses and Preferences for Outcomes and Risks of Treatments (SUPPORT). *JAMA* 274(20):1591-8.

Teno, J.M., Clarridge B.R., Casey V., Welch, L.C., Wetle, T., Shield, R., and Mor, V. (2004) Family perspectives on end-of-life care at the last place of care. *JAMA* 291(1):88-93.

The last Acts Coalition, *means to a better end: a report on dying in America today.* (2002) Washington DC: Partnership for Caring. www.lastacts.org.

Townsend, J., Frank, A.O., Femount, D., Dyer, S., Karran, O., Walgrove, A., and Piper, M. (1990) Terminal cancer and patients' preferences for place of death, a prospective study, *BMJ.* 301(6749):415-417.

5
The Role of Cancer Rehabilitation in the Maintenance of Functional Integrity and Quality of Life

Andrea Cheville MD, Vivek Khemka MB BCh BAO, and Sean O'Mahony MB BCh BAO

1. Introduction

Rehabilitation too often remains clinically marginalized in the care of cancer patients. The perception that only patients capable of full community and vocational pursuits with unrestricted life spans stand to benefit from rehabilitation is inaccurate. Although physical medicine and rehabilitation, or physiatry, was initially dedicated to transitioning individuals with anatomically devastating injuries back to productive lives, the field has broadened considerably. This increased scope is a response to medical advances that have radically altered the prognoses of many formerly fatal diseases. Integration of rehabilitation services in the care of patients with far-advanced pulmonary and cardiac disease is standard. Comparable services are rarely offered to cancer patients, even in the early stages of disease. The purpose of rehabilitation as outlined in this chapter is to improve the quality of life irrespective of etiology or anticipated survival.

The number and severity of functional impairments correlate with disability among cancer patients (Cheville, 2002). As disease progresses, impairments become increasingly common. Most patients develop multiple deficits in the advanced stages of cancer. For example, patients with advanced breast cancer develop conjointly chemotherapy-induced peripheral neuropathies, lymphedema and steroid myopathies, referring to injury to peripheral nerves, edema or swelling secondary to injury in lymphatic channels, and muscle injury associated with use of steroids, respectively. Also plexopathies, or injury to the nerve plexus or network of nerve fibers that pass from one peripheral nerve to

ANDREA CHEVILLE • Mayo Clinic Department of Rehabilitation Medicine, Rochester MA. VIVEK KHEMKA • Palliative Care Fellow, Palliative Care Service, Montefiore Medical Center, Bronx, NY, USA. SEAN O'MAHONY • Montefiore Medical Center, Albert Einstein College of Medicine, Bronx, NY, USA, 111 E. 210th Street, Bronx 10467.

another. Patients' capacity to negotiate each additional impairment diminishes with waning functional reserve. Eventually their ability to functionally compensate is exhausted leading to severe disability and loss of autonomy.

Particular impairments are associated with abrupt functional decline in the absence of rehabilitation. Pleural or pulmonary compromise can acutely undermine aerobic reserve leading to severe exertional intolerance. Malignant lesions, particularly osseous or bone metastases, can undermine the essential supporting structures of the musculoskeletal system. Often abnormal and ultimately dysfunctional biomechanical movement patterns result. Patients with lower extremity sarcomas undergoing limb salvage procedures are an excellent example. Substantial portions of the knee and hip extensor muscles may be resected. If patients are to resume independent ambulation, intact muscles must be aggressively strengthened and biomechanical patterns modified through concerted physical therapy. Nonsurgical anticancer treatments, including radiation therapy and chemotherapy, can also injure nerves and muscles. Essentially, compromise of any cardiopulmonary or musculoskeletal structure has the potential to produce severe disability. The potential is greatest among cancer patients with pre-existing medical and functional morbidity.

Classically, rehabilitation focuses on reducing the level of disability and handicap associated with particular impairments. Impairments most commonly remediated are those due to neurological or musculoskeletal injuries. An extensive literature describes the effectiveness of established interventions in improving function in affected patients. For example, severe motor deficits associated with paraplegia can be mitigated through the prescription of an appropriate wheelchair, instruction in independent transfer techniques, and use of assistive devices for the performance of activities of daily living (ADLs). Little of the rehabilitation literature relates specifically to cancer patients, However, a growing number of case series suggest that conventional approaches are equally effective in remediating cancer related impairments. Marciniak and associates at Northwestern University studied patients admitted to a rehabilitation hospital because of functional loss related to cancer or its treatment over a two-year period. With rehabilitation, significant functional gains were made between admission and discharge in all subgroups. The presence of metastatic disease did not diminish benefits. (Marciniak *et al.*, 1996)

Functional decline has an erosive effect on cancer patients' psychological well being (Breitbart, 2000; Natterlund *et al.*, 2000). Dependence for mobility and self-care is associated with diminished quality of life among chronically ill patients. A fundamental rehabilitation approach involves instructing patients in compensatory strategies for mobility and the performance of ADLs. By deconstructing tasks into discrete steps, therapists can determine which step(s) in a task sequence patients are unable to execute or produce pain. Intact physiological systems and adaptive equipment substitute for impaired structures restoring patients' autonomy. Qualitative reports of cancer rehabilitation programs that this approach can meaningfully enhance function among cancer patients, even those with far advanced disease (Yoshioka, 1994).

Failure to optimize functional integrity throughout the continuum of illness may limit cancer patients' access to effective disease modifying therapies. Poor performance status renders patients ineligible for some chemotherapy regimens and clinical trials. In addition, cancer-associated disability is a source of substantially increased expenditures for patients, their caregivers, and their health care providers. Many of the described modalities are reported to be effective and economically viable.

2. Epidemiology of Functional Deficits

With the availability of more effective anti-neoplastic therapies patients with cancer are living for longer periods of time. The five-year survival rate for breast cancer, for example, currently exceeds 85%. Enhanced survival however is often accompanied by reduced functioning and health-related quality of life. Concern over loss of the capacity for self-determined movement and activity is very common among patients with advanced cancer. Axelson et al., in Sweden, found that in the last six weeks of life most quality-of-life ratings correlated with "the ability to do what one wants, physical strength, and a sense of meaningfulness" (Axelsson). Diminished functioning can be as feared as pain, and a source of profound psychological distress. In fact fear of "becoming a burden" is the number one reason that patients request euthanasia (Willems et al., 2000). The rapidly aging population will result in greater numbers of elderly cancer patients living for extended periods with progressive dependency.

Limited data suggest that rehabilitation services are underutilized among patients with metastatic cancer. A study of patients with stage IV breast cancer receiving chemotherapy at Memorial Sloan Kettering Cancer Center demonstrated significant functional deterioration and loss of vocational viability. There were 533 measurable functional impairments in 170 patients. However fewer than 20% had received an intervention geared toward functional restoration. Two thirds of patients who were working at the time of stage IV diagnosis lost their jobs as a consequence of cancer-related pain and impairments. Only 1% of the study cohort who were not working at the time of stage IV diagnosis subsequently became employed despite widespread interest in joining the work force (Cheville, 2002).

Joann Lynn and her colleagues have devised a paradigm to characterize the trajectories of functional decline in cancer and other illnesses. There is a long period perhaps over several years during which functional capacity remains almost at baseline with several episodes of decline in response to disease progression, recurrence or major isease modifying therapies such as surgery, radiation or chemotherapy. The final phase in advanced disease is often characterized by a dramatic drop off in functioning in the final months of life with marked physical dependency (Lynn and Adamson, 2003). This enables oncologists to identify patients who are eligible for hospice referral based on a physician estimate of life expectancy of six months or less. This perhaps accounts for the preponderance of cancer as a leading diagnosis for up to

70% of hospice patients until comparatively recently and up to 50% of cancer patients receiving hospice care. Given that cancer is usually a disease of the elderly, functional reserve can be anticipated to be lessened by medical comorbidities. Many such patients can be anticipated to have pre existent diabetic neuropathies, congestive heart failure, cognitive deficits and degenerative arthritic disorders. All of the above renders patients more vulnerable to cancer-related impairments, and more likely to develop severe impairments. Also patients with co morbid illnesses are less able to compensate for new impairments and therefore at increased risk of significant disability.

3. Performance Status and Survival

The presence of functional deficits has long been recognized by oncologists as being predictive of survival and response to treatment. Physical performance has also been found to be predictive of survival in patients with advanced disease and is used as an eligibility criterion for hospice enrollment in the US. An assessment of functional status must be incorporated into the decision making process when considering the use of palliative chemotherapy or radiation. Patients with persistently reduced levels of functioning can be anticipated to have much higher risks of treatment toxicity and lower likelihood of treatment response. As many cancer patients continue to receive cytotoxic treatments within days or weeks of death in the US, it is of central importance that standardized assessments of performance status be incorporated into initial and follow-up evaluations of such patients.

The Karnofsky Performance Status (KPS) measure was developed in the 1940's and is one of the most familiar scales to clinicians caring for cancer patients. The Eastern Cooperative Oncology Group (ECOG) Scale is another commonly used measure in research and clinical practice. Scores on this measure are predictive of survival in patients with advanced cancer (Karnofsky, 1949; Buccheri et al., 1996; Loprinzi et al., 1994). In a population of cancer patients enrolled in a rehabilitation program with a physician prediction of survival of 3-12 months a KPS score of less than 50 was associated with short survival. Patients with higher KPS generally lived for longer and patients in the last 2 months of life had a rapid drop off in KPS. The National Hospice Study of over 1000 patients admitted to hospice in the 1980's suggested that for every decile increase in KPS score survival increased by 2 weeks (Yates et al., 1980; Mor et al., 1984).

But the widely known KPS and ECOG scales may lack sensitivity to detect important changes in functioning in patients with advanced disease. The scores for many patients in palliative care settings tend to cluster in the lower deciles (O'Mahony et al., 2005). An increasing number of scales have been developed for use in palliative care settings such as the Palliative Performance Scale (PPS) and the Edmonton Functional Assessment Tool (EFAT). (Kaasa and Wessel, 2001; Anderson et al., 1996). These scales are used by nurses in home hospice, inpatient palliative care units and hospice unit settings. These scales are predictive of short term survival. For example, all patients admitted to a hospice unit with PPS scores of 10 died with an average survival of 1.9 days in contrast to patients with scores of 40 or higher. Forty-four percent of the latter group survived to discharge.

The scales cited above are sensitive to the presence of high levels of disability but do not assist with identification of the cause of disability. Assessment scales that are more commonly reported in the physical medicine literature include the Modified Barthel Index (MBI) and the Functional Independence Measure (FIM) (Hamilton et al., 1987; Mahoney and Barthel, 1965; Granger et al., 1979).

The incorporation of more sensitive performance scales into clinical practice may improve outcomes in a number of ways. It will enable caregivers to provide patients and families with more precise, and evidence-based estimates of survival time. Palliative care providers will be better able to distinguish between patients with very short survival times who may die within hours, and those patients expected to survive for more than 10 days. In the latter group transfer from an acute to a sub-acute facility is a reasonable option. Whereas transferring the former group could subject patients, their families and their professional caregivers to needless trauma. Data garnered from application of these scales may also help health care administrators to anticipate bed availability and staffing requirements in palliative settings. The ability of these scales to detect subtle shifts in functional status may enable them to more accurately gauge the impact of palliative chemotherapy.

4. Quality of Life and Functional Impairment in Cancer

Cancer treatment planning is increasingly including functional status and quality of life as essential outcomes. According to a study by members of the Veterans Affairs Laryngeal Cancer Study Group, patients whose treatment left the larynx intact had better quality-of-life scores compared to those who underwent surgical laryngectomy. Better scores in the chemotherapy plus radiation therapy group appeared to be related to more freedom from pain, emotional well-being and lower levels of depression, rather than preservation of speech functions (Terrell et al., 1998; Larto, 1990; Weymuller et al., 2000).

Why do some terminal cancer patients choose hastened death? Desire for hastened death is stronger in patients with reduced mobility and physical functioning. Patients fear becoming dependent, losing control, developing urinary or fecal incontinence, and having to forsake their familial and social roles.

O'Mahony and associates studied 131 newly referred patients to the Pain and Palliative Care Service at Memorial Sloan Kettering Cancer Center or newly admitted to Calvary Hospital in New York. Desire for hastened death scores were correlated with depression, low social support, poor spiritual well-being and cancer pain. According to the results improvement in depression scores appeared to be a major factor in moderating desire for hastened death. Intensive pain management had less influence on desire for hastened death. Breitbart and colleagues at Memorial Sloan Kettering Cancer Center and Calvary Hospital analyzed desire for hastened death in 92 terminally ill cancer patients receiving palliative care. Nearly two thirds of patients who were identified as having depression or hopelessness with the study measures had a high desire for hastened death. Among those who were neither depressed nor hopeless, none had a high desire for hastened death (O'Mahony et al., 2005; Breitbart et al., 2000).

Cancer patients remain keenly interested in receiving rehabilitation services while manifesting psychological distress from their cancer associated functional deficits. In a study of patients with stage IV breast cancer by Cheville and associates, patients' levels of distress were highly correlated with KPS scores of 40 to 50, a score of 40 indicates that a person has high levels of disability and needs special care. Virtually all patients with KPS scores between 40 and 70 expressed very strong interest in receiving physical therapy (Cheville, 2002).

A plethora of multidimensional quality of life instruments have been developed for cancer studies and those in use in other settings are commonly used. The European Organization for Research and Treatment of Cancer (EORTC QLQ-C30) instrument for example has been used in over 1,500 studies worldwide (Aaronson et al., 1993). The incorporation of these multi-dimensional instruments enables the identification of concerning treatment toxicities and functional deficits that would formerly have remained unde-tected. Instruments such as the Functional Assessment of Cancer Treatment (FACT G) examine multiple domains of functioning: social, familial, physi-cal, emotional and spiritual well-being have been further adapted to specific cancers (Cella et al., 1996). Domain-specific measures evaluate prevalent symptoms such as pain, fatigue, anxiety and depression (Loge and Kaasa, 1998; Endicott, 1983; Spielberger, 1983; Cleeland and Ryan, 1983; Zigmond and Snaith, 1983).

Other multidimensional assessment tools such as the The Memorial Symptom Assessment Scale Short form (MSAS-SF) evaluate multiple symptoms and include global distress subscales (Chang et al., 2000). More recently developed quality-of-life measures for palliative care settings include the Schedule for the Evaluation of Individual Quality-of-Life questionnaire (SEIQoL). This instru-ment enables patients to nominate important domains of functioning and then to assess their level of functioning in that domain. It is available in an abbrevi-ated format which enhances its utility in medically ill patients. However in general the development of such tools has tended to occur in non-terminally ill populations. Scales such as the Missoula- VITAS quality-of-life index developed for use in the hospice care setting may not be acceptable for patients who are chronically ill with life-threatening illnesses but who have not accepted limited life expectancy (Waldron et al., 1999; Byock and Merriman, 1998).

End-of-life researchers are well advised to limit research questionnaire burden in acknowledgement of patients' limited physical reserves. However, inclusion of outcomes that only address single domains or symptoms may not adequately characterize the impact of a particular intervention. Reductions in individual symptom severity, notably pain, that do not directly associate with global satisfaction or health-related quality-of-life may reflect a response shift. For example, patients may reframe their functioning and quality-of- life expectations, or develop other potentially distressing losses and symptoms (O'Mahony *et al.*, 2005; Hearn and Higginson, 1999).

5. Efficacy of Cancer Rehabilitation

An increasing body of evidence supports the effectiveness of interdisciplinary cancer rehabilitation. Yoshioka and associates in Japan, reported results of physical therapy in a series of terminal patients admitted to an inpatient hospice. The Barthel Mobility Index was chosen as the primary outcome measure. There was substantial improvement in BMI scores (mean 27% increase) following completion of physical therapy. Of significance forty-six of the 301 patients achieved sufficient autonomy for home discharge. A prospective descriptive study of over 800 patients reported significant improvements in functional status and quality-of-life for a wide range of cancer-related impairments (Lehman *et al.*, 1978). Other studies as early as the 1970s demonstrate impressive improvements in functional integrity measuring outcomes such as return to "mainstream life" in between 47% and 80% of patients. A more recent series of patients who were admitted for in patient rehabilitation resulted in an increase in the proportion of patients capable of independent ambulation from 10% to 56%. Despite this growing evidence base, integrated specialist rehabilitation services continue to be the exception rather than the rule in the care of most patients. The potential benefits of rehabilitation modalities extend to hospice settings (Lehman *et al.*, 1978; Mellette, 1977; Dietz, 1974; Harvey *et al.*, 1982; Yoshioka, 1994).

Fatigue is now understood to be the most common symptom associated with cancer and its treatment. In a study by Dimeo and associates, in Germany, patients with advanced cancer receiving high-dose chemotherapy followed by peripheral blood stem cell transplantation carried out an exercise training program during hospitalization. The program consisted of biking on an ergometer in the supine position for 30 minutes daily. By the time of hospital discharge, fatigue and somatic complaints had increased significantly in the control group but not in the training group. Moreover by the time of hospital discharge, the training group had a significant improvement in several scores of psychological distress (eg. obsessive-compulsive traits, fear and phobic anxiety). This was not observed in the control group. In another study, Dimeo and associates evaluated the effects of an endurance training program shortly after patients completed high-dose chemotherapy. Treadmill exercise (30 minutes daily for six weeks) contributed to improved performance status and reduced fatigue in the training group but not the controls (Dimeo *et al.*, 1997).

6. Development of Rehabilitation Goals

Rehabilitation goals should reflect patient age, type and stage of malignancy, medical morbidities, baseline fitness level and education. Dietz developed an approach to rehabilitative goal setting for cancer patients in which he defined four complementary, and interrelated, yet distinct types of function-oriented interventions (Dietz, 1980). These include restorative, supportive, preventative and palliative rehabilitative interventions.

Restorative rehabilitation has as its goal the return of the patient to his or her premorbid level of functioning when no lasting impairment is anticipated. Such approaches are often utilized following intensive anti-cancer treatments. For example, after mastectomy, restorative approaches can restore shoulder range of motion and upper extremity strength. Structured progressive aerobic conditioning represents a very effective restorative technique for patients undergoing bone marrow transplantation. It can allow them to recover their premorbid fitness levels. In contrast, supportive rehabilitation attempts to optimize functioning in patients with permanent impairments. An example of this approach would include the multimodal techniques used to rehabilitate patients after limb salvage procedures such as internal hemi-pelvectomy (this procedure is limb-sparing but often requires removing the top of the femur, hip joint and most of the pelvis on the effected side). Combined interventions focused on enhancement of proprioception, balance and ambulatory patterns can successfully compensate for impaired limb and pelvic biomechanics. Proprioception is also called the sixth sense, referring to the individual's unconscious perception of movement of muscles, tendons and the joints.

Preventative approaches attempt to preclude impairments due to cancer or cancer directed therapies. Examples of this approach include prophylactic range of motion exercises to reduce radiation-induced soft tissue contractures. Education of caregivers is often a highly effective preventative approach. Empowering and informing caregivers can help reduce predictable complications such as skin ulcers that result from immobility and chemotherapeutic neuropathies.

Palliative rehabilitation encompasses supportive approaches designed to reduce patients' dependence in mobility and self care activities. Emotional support and comfort are concurrently provided. For example, preservation of autonomous bowel and bladder continence is an important palliative goal in cancer patients with advanced disease. The presence of incontinence predicts profound psychological distress. Simple rehabilitative interventions can often extend patients ability to toilet independently till the very terminal stages of cancer (King *et al.*, 1994; Hillel and Patten, 1990; Ko *et al.*, 1998; Cheville, 2005). Anasarca (generalized edema) and progressive lymphedema are common among end-stage cancer patients. Palliative rehabilitation approaches such as lymphatic drainage techniques and multi-layer compression bandaging can minimize edema, thereby enhancing patient comfort and mobility. Additionally, these measures function preventatively to reduce the likelihood of local skin breakdown and infections.

7. Rehabilitation Interventions

Rehabilitative interventions can be grouped into seven principal categories. These include physical modalities, compensatory strategies, use of assistive devices, therapeutic exercise, environmental modification, use of orthotics and cargiver education. All interventions share the underlying goal of facilitating safe and maximally autonomous function. Frequently, interventions from each category are combined and integrated into an individualized rehabilitation plan. Cancer patients' reliance on different interventions can be expected to change over time contingent on the evolution of their disease.

In the present context, the term "modalities" refers to physical agents used to achieve specific soft tissue effects. Modalities should be used to realize discrete clinical goals such as reduction of muscle spasms or joint contractures. Thermal modalities are widely accessible and commonly utilized. Therapeutic cold inhibits nociception (experience of pain), reduces collagen extensibility, and retards nerve conduction. Unfortunately, cooling modalities often cause discomfort at the temperatures and treatment durations required for biophysiological efficacy. In the absence of local inflammation, strong patient preference, or other compelling indications, therapeutic cold should be avoided in advanced cancer. The muscle relaxant effects of heat make it highly effective in alleviating pain from spasms. Such spasms occur commonly over bone metastases and at other sites of tumor invasion. Care must be taken when heat is applied to skin with compromised sensation. Topical heat comes in many forms including hydrocollator packs, heat lamps, heating pads, etc. Moist, conductive heat will be transferred most efficiently. Deep heating modalities such as ultrasound and short wave diathermy are seldom indicated in the management of cancer-related impairments. In the author's experience however, severe radiation-induced fibrosis can be reduced more successfully when ultrasound is conservatively combined with conventional manual techniques.

Massage in its many forms falls within the rubric of physical modalities. Fundamentally benign, it is rare that massage fails to benefit cancer patients if only through the calming effects of human touch. The rationale for massage should be clarified. Determination of its efficacy will depend on whether it is enlisted nonspecifically to enhance patient well being, or in a concerted effort to address a discrete problem. Many specialized massage techniques have been developed to affect specific anatomic structures and pathophysiological processes. For example, *manual lymphatic drainage* enhances lymphatic function, while *myofascial release techniques* alleviate trigger points for pain and excessive muscle tone. Many physical therapists use massage techniques in conjunction with other rehabilitative techniques to potentiate functional outcomes.

Instructing patients in compensatory strategies is a cornerstone of both occupational and physical therapy. Occupational therapists generally focus their attention on the fine motor coordination and task sequencing required for ADL performance. In contrast, physical therapists address gross mobility issues such as transfers (eg. from bed to chair), ambulation, and climbing stairs. By deconstructing activities to their finest component steps, therapists can identify steps that are undermined by pain, weakness, or coordination deficits. Alternative ways of executing the affected task sequence are then provided. Such compensatory strategies can significantly extend patients' autonomy in all functional domains.

When impairments undermine the execution of ADL or mobility task sequences, assistive devices can be used to compensate. A wide variety of assistive devices are available to allow independent grooming, dressing and feeding. Occupational therapists help patients select appropriate devices and efficiently incorporate them into task sequences. Simple dressing aids like "button holers," "sockers," and long-handled shoe horns can preserve the independence of patients with severe chemotherapeutic neuropathies. Assistive devices for ambulation range from rolling platform walkers to standard canes. Patients often adopt devices discarded by friends or family members. This practice should be discouraged unless supervised by a physical therapist. Physical therapists are expert in evaluating patients' needs. By watching patients ambulate with different devices, therapists can select the device that allows safe and maximally efficient gait.

Cancer patients may have motor deficits of such severity that assistive devices must supply all power for mobility. Examples include motorized wheelchairs, scooters and Hoyer lifts. The patient's prognoses should be considered in the acquisition of these potentially costly devices. Often rental units are available. Although expensive, the benefits of sustaining patients' community integration and social spheres through preserved mobility are immeasurable.

Therapeutic exercise to enhance aerobic conditioning, strength, coordination, and flexibility comprises an integral part of rehabilitation. Therapeutic exercise exploits the body's capacity to adapt dynamically to imposed demands. For example, muscles increase in bulk and power output when they are successively brought to the point of failure. Patients with advanced cancer are seldom deemed candidates for therapeutic exercise. The fallacy of this reasoning lies partially in the misperception that exercise must be rigorous and sustained to have meaningful benefit. Modest, brief exercise can prevent and reverse progressive deconditioning. Most research on exercise in cancer has looked at the effect of aerobic exercise on functional capacity, symptom burden and quality of life. Several investigations have demonstrated significant benefit with respect to fatigue, functional status, pain, and nausea when aerobic conditioning is administered concurrently with adjuvant chemotherapy for breast cancer, or after high-dose chemotherapy during bone marrow transplantation (Winningham et al., 1994; Dimeo et al., 1997). As yet little empiric information is available to guide the use of exercise in advanced cancer. However, the successful use of resistive exercise to enhance function among cachetic patients with advanced AIDS argues that conventional techniques will not harm most patients (O'Brien *et al.*, 2004(a); O'Brien *et al.*, 2004(b)).

All cancer patients whose functional decline arises from impaired strength or stamina are excellent candidates for therapeutic exercise. When patients are medically stable, exercise can begin with gentle active and active-assisted twice-daily ranging of the extremities. Brief isometric muscle contractions can be performed in bed against gravity or with gravity eliminated. Isometric or static contractions are those involving no angular motion of the joint on which the muscle acts. Therabands can be tied to a patient's bed rails and bedroom furniture to provide resistance for isotonic exercise. Isotonic exercise, involves constant tone as muscles move through their entire contractile range. Isotonics are preferred since they strengthen muscle at all joint angles within the functional range.

Cancer patients are particularly prone to disruption of physical therapy because of unanticipated hospitalizations and competing medical appointments. Every time a disruption occurs approval must be obtained from payers for resumption of therapy. The integration of physical medicine teams into all phases of cancer disease management systems could reduce some of these interruptions.

Environmental modification offers many patients the opportunity to remain at home in the face of progressive disability. Typical modifications allow independent access into the home and increase home safety. Installation of ramps or lifts permits wheelchair bound patients to enter dwellings elevated from street level. Stairglides allow plegic patients to negotiate two-level homes. Rails and grab bars can be installed in virtually any part of the home to ensure safe mobility. Durable medical equipment such as raised toilet seats, commodes, and tub benches offer a relatively inexpensive means of maximizing safety and independence during bathing and toileting.

Orthotics are braces designed to alter joint mechanics compromised by weak muscles, pain, impaired sensation, bone metastases, or disrupted anatomical integrity. Orthotics are highly versatile and can facilitate a variety of therapeutic goals. Orthotics can restore alignment, protect vulnerable structures, stretch soft tissue contractures, substitute for weak muscles, or stabilize joints in positions of least pain. However, use of orthotics for cancer patients must be tempered by the overarching mandate of patient comfort. For example, a molded body jacket would provide maximal stability for a patient with diffuse vertebral metastases. However, the discomfort associated with wearing such devices, as well as the difficulty putting them on and off, makes their use unfeasible for many advanced cancer patients. Similarly, Dynasplint® produces orthotics designed to apply steady pressure on joints in order to elongate contracted soft tissue. Although soft tissue contractures are common among cancer patients, the expense and discomfort associated with Dynasplint® use must be carefully considered before use in advanced cancer patients. It is important to communicate each patient's prognosis, goals of treatment, financial resources, and symptom control issues to the occupational therapist or orthotist responsible for splint fabrication. This increases the likelihood that patients will receive an orthotic suited to their unique requirements.

Education of caregivers is a vital and often overlooked dimension of comprehensive rehabilitation. Most caregivers will shoulder increasing responsibility as patients' become progressively disabled. It is critical that caregivers receive instruction on how to protect themselves from musculoskeletal strain. Simple guidance in body mechanics can enhance the ease and safety with which caregivers transfer patients. Instruction in modalities such as topical heat, massage, and the application of compression offer caregivers a means of contributing to symptom control.

8. Precautions in Cancer Rehabilitation

A climate of exaggerated caution too often limits cancer rehabilitation. Specific therapeutic precautions reflect a fear of injuring patients, or worse, spreading their cancer. While it is important to appreciate that cancer patients are predisposed to a host of adverse complications (e.g. hemorrhage, disease progression), it is equally important to recognize that a causal relationship has not been established between such complications and physiatric interventions. Inactivity causes far greater long-term difficulty for the majority of cancer patients. At present, no precautions are supported by empirical data. Often they reinforce ambivalence toward structured, incremental physical activity.

Leukopenia and thrombocytopenia, respectfully an insufficiency of circulating white blood cells and an insufficiency of blood platelets, commonly occur following the administration of chemotherapy. There are inconsistent guidelines limiting physical activity in the face of chemotherapy-induced cytopenias. Existing precautions are arbitrary, and lack empirical testing. None have been shown to limit adverse events. Leukopenia is of less concern than thrombocytopenia, given the associated risk of intracranial hemorrhage or uncontrolled bleeding after a fall. Among National Cancer Institute designated comprehensive cancer centers, cut-off platelet counts below which physical therapy is contraindicated range from 25K to no lower limit. No differences between institutions in the incidence of spontaneous hemorrhage have been detected. Patients undergoing allo- and autogeneic bone marrow transplants typically spend 7-21 days with platelets counts of 5-12 thousand. During this interval, most patients perform all ADLS independently, ambulate, transfer, and lift >10 lbs repeatedly without hemorrhage. When spontaneous bleeding does occur, it is typically not associated with physical activity. Given the routinely well-tolerated levels of physical activity in severely thrombocytopenic patients, reconsideration of current precautions is warranted. Overzealous imposition of restrictions on physical therapy and exercise in this population can lead to rapid deconditioning, bone demineralization, thrombosis and formation of contractures.

Rehabilitation is an essential component of an integrated pain management program geared toward symptom control and autonomous function. Palliative care providers often are trained to manage pain and other symptoms in bed-bound patients. If the delivery of symptom-oriented treatment is integrated with patient mobilization, quality-of-life can be enhanced by a focus on strategies that enhance function.

9. Venues for Rehabilitation Service Delivery

Rehabilitation services are traditionally provided at five different sites. These include acute hospital wards, inpatient rehabilitation units, skilled nursing facilities, patients' homes, and outpatient physical and occupational therapy clinics. The strengths and limitations of the care delivered at these different sites varies considerably. Familiarity with the distinctions between them is critical for appropriate rehabilitation referrals. Access to each site requires a specific sequence of referrals and/or approvals.

Delivery of rehabilitation services on acute hospital wards requires a formal consult from the primary service. Too often such requests are made far into a patient's hospital course after severe functional deterioration has occurred. Timely involvement of rehabilitation services requires that a forward-thinking primary team member recognize the need for functional preservation soon after admission. Some departments, recognizing the critical contribution that rehabilitation staff makes to positive outcomes, have incorporated physical therapy and occupational therapy into the critical care pathways for specific patient populations. Reports of such efforts have demonstrated medical and financial benefits (Tiep, 1997). Once consulted, physiatrists or therapists are integral in determining patients' rehabilitation needs at the time of discharge. The rehabilitation consultant can assist in determining the level of care after hospital discharge.

Access to inpatient rehabilitation units requires transfer following an acute hospital stay. Occasionally outpatients are directly admitted to inpatient units if sufficient need can be demonstrated. Whether and where patients receive inpatient rehabilitation depends on the efforts of hospital social workers and discharge planners. The assessment of a rehabilitation consultant and the approval of third party payers may also be required. Patients are accepted at the discretion of the inpatient units' admission departments. If defensible rehabilitation goals or a realistic discharge plan cannot be established, access will often be denied. Patterns of referral to rehabilitation vary across institutions, diagnoses, and caregivers.

Many of the same factors determine access to home rehabilitation services. Home rehabilitation services are generally initiated following discharge from an acute hospital ward or inpatient rehabilitation unit. The involvement of home services must be formally solicited at the time of discharge. Patients can also receive home rehabilitation services through visiting nurse referrals. If a nurse notes that a patient is unsafe or functionally impaired, he or she can request a home physical therapy or occupational therapy evaluation. This is fortunate since visiting nurses represent one of the most common and reliable avenues by which cancer patients receive rehabilitation services. Therapists are responsible for requesting other rehabilitation services as appropriate, such as speech therapy. Third party payers rarely offer significant opposition to the initiation of home services due to the reduced cost. However continuation of services for any length of time can require ongoing justification and formidable amounts of paperwork.

Most cancer outpatients receive rehabilitation services at free-standing or hospital-affiliated PT and OT clinics. Reimbursement requires a professional caretaker's prescription. Patients who are unable to obtain a prescription can pay out of pocket for services but this option is often prohibitively expensive. Optimal outcomes require that oncologists recognize and promote the benefits of outpatient rehabilitation. Patients who lack their oncologists' full endorsement may not attend therapy sessions or fully embrace rehabilitation goals. Since routine oncological care is not functionally oriented, clinicians may lack sufficient familiarity with PT and OT to appropriately refer their patients in a timely manner. This may partially account for the underutilization of outpatient rehabilitation services by cancer patients.

The different sites of rehabilitation care delivery have unique attributes which may or may not be suited to a specific patient. The strengths and weaknesses of each venue are discussed in the following paragraphs beginning with inpatient rehabilitation units. Inpatient units fall into three categories based on the breadth and intensity of available services. Acute, subacute, and skilled nursing facility (SNF) levels of rehabilitation offer incrementally fewer hours of therapy per day. For reimbursement, inpatient rehabilitation facilities (IRF) must provide a minimum of three hours of physical and occupational therapy per day. IRFs also offer many additional services such as neuropsychological counseling, speech therapy, prosthetics, orthotics, and recreational therapy. IRFs are intended to offer patients with severe, remediable impairments an opportunity to receive concentrated services that would otherwise be inaccessible. These facilities commonly admit patients after severe injuries affecting major neurological structures. Several retrospective chart reviews found that cancer patients admitted to IRFs achieve the same rate of functional recovery as patients with comparable impairments due to trauma or ischemia (Garman et al., 2004; Teichmann, 2002).

Admissions to IRFs are costly. Third party payers regularly scrutinize patients' progress to ensure that they consistently improve and meet their rehabilitation goals. If patients fail to attend therapy sessions or to derive benefit, payers can deny or reduce reimbursement. Despite findings to the contrary cancer patients are considered more prone to develop medical morbidities and to miss therapy sessions as a result (Coleman *et al.*, 2003; Oldervall *et al.*, 2004; Pickett *et al.*, 2002; Friendenreich and Courneya, 1996). This biases the medical directors of some IRFs against cancer-related admissions. Ideally those patients' with realistic goals that warrant intensive rehabilitation should be admitted to acute units irrespective of their diagnoses. Short, targeted rehabilitation stays can reduce the chance of unplanned acute readmissions due to caretaker overload. Justifiable goals for debilitated cancer patients can include provision with appropriate equipment and family education. Careful review of patients' needs and capacity to benefit from services will reduce the likelihood of a mismatch between patient status and level of care. Such mismatches lead to dissatisfaction on all fronts. Excessive rehabilitation demands can aggravate the distress of already taxed cancer patients.

Subacute and SNF levels of inpatient rehabilitation impose fewer therapeutic demands on patients. Subacute units provide a minimum of two hours of PT/OT services per day while SNF units provide only one hour. During the reduced therapy time subacute and SNF units offer less physically demanding treatments. They often lack the special equipment that acute units routinely offer such as standing frames, suspended harnesses, and exercise machines. Speech therapy and neuropsychological counseling are rarely available. Patients who are too debilitated for home discharge, but unable to tolerate three hours of therapy per day, are generally transferred to subacute and SNF units. Such units can provide enough structured activity to prevent deconditioning while patients recover sufficient independence for safe home discharge.

IRFs can be free-standing, or near or within an acute care hospital. An important consideration in transferring cancer patients with complex medical issues is the availability of specialized clinical services. In general it is always preferable that cancer patients go to units housed near or within large secondary or tertiary medical centers offering a broad range of consultative expertise. Oncologists and palliative medical teams can often provide uninterrupted care despite patients' change in location. The presence of familiar caregivers provides invaluable reassurance to patients, particularly when confronted by the demands of rehabilitation. IRFs within hospitals offer patients the option of receiving chemotherapy or radiation while participating in rehabilitation. Access to a large institutional pharmacy offers patients access to a wider range of analgesics and expertise in parenteral (injectable) delivery systems. Units within hospitals are generally more willing to accept cancer patients with parenteral or epidural PCA pumps. The assistance of specialty consultants increases the likelihood that medical complications will be successfully managed on the rehabilitation ward. In freestanding facilities, patients who develop even minor problems may be transferred back to acute care. Such transfers interrupt rehabilitative efforts and are highly disruptive for patients.

Home physical or occupational therapy has the distinct advantage of offering rehabilitation services in the environment where patients must function.

A disadvantage is the lack of specialized equipment, therapeutic expertise and, at times, adequate space. In general, home physical or occupational therapists visit patients' homes two to three times per week. The goals of treatment are quite basic; independent transfers, ambulation, and climbing stairs. Equipment and family education are incorporated as appropriate. Once patients achieve sufficient autonomy for safe household-level mobility and ADL performance, therapy is discontinued. Patients may be provided with a strengthening or stretching program of limited intensity. Home-based rehabilitation does not equip patients for community mobility, higher-level ADL performance, or vocational reintegration. Patients are seldom referred for more challenging outpatient services after termination. The lack of referral to higher levels of care is appropriate in far advanced disease when patients' maximal potential rarely exceeds the basic requirements of household functioning. However, all cancer patients should not be dismissed as being unable to benefit from more rigorous outpatient therapy.

Outpatient rehabilitation services are generally delivered to "well" patients with discrete musculoskeletal or neurological problems. Though many cancer patients can benefit from outpatient PT or OT, failure to consider their unique needs creates the real possibility of causing harm. Indiscriminate application of routine treatment algorithms to cancer patients can undermine rather than enhance well-being. The fact that few therapists have cultivated expertise with cancer-related impairments remains a barrier to optimal outcomes. Nonetheless outpatient rehabilitation offers tremendous advantages. Most facilities are equipped with highly specialized equipment that permits formulation of individually tailored treatment regimens. Balance enhancing machines for vestibular rehabilitation are an example. In addition, the high patient volume typical of outpatient facilities allows therapists to subspecialize. Lymphedema, pelvic floor, upper extremity, and neuro-rehabilitation services offer unique treatments that cannot be feasibly delivered in other settings.

Financial and logistical barriers can represent a significant threat to the delivery of outpatient services. Transportation poses an obstacle for many patients. While patients regularly travel to receive anti-cancer therapies, their willingness may not extend to rehabilitation services. This is particularly true when travel represents a significant out of pocket expense. Increasing therapy co-payments presents another financial barrier. Many third party payers require co-payments of more than US$25 per therapy session. For financially depleted patients, the cost associated with an 8-session therapy course may be untenable. Capitation presents an additional challenge, particularly when patients require specialty services. Patients belonging to health maintenance organizations are 'capitated' to a particular therapy site contingent on the affiliation of their primary care provider. If the capitation site does not offer the required therapy service, special, and at time laborious, approval must be obtained or patients are faced with formidable costs. Once initiated, continued outpatient therapy requires ongoing third party payer approvals. Obtaining approval depends entirely on the diligence, motivation, and skill of the treating therapist.

Despite the many venues for rehabilitation care delivery, available data indicate that disconcertingly few cancer patients receive any functional remediation. This is unfortunate in light of the growing evidence demonstrating that conventional rehabilitation interventions are efficacious in cancer populations.

10. Barriers to Rehabilitation

Despite the high prevalence of functional deficits during the treatment of cancer, access to comprehensive rehabilitative services remains the exception rather than the norm. Impediments to effective rehabilitation span institutional-, caregiver-, patient- and society-based barriers. Rehabilitation professionals are rarely integrated into oncological teams that plan therapy and supervise the care of cancer patients. Referral to rehabilitation providers is often reactive in response to periods of abrupt functional decline, e.g. the perioperative period. Often rehabilitation services are solicited at the end of an acute hospital stay to fulfill disposition requirements. Many cancer patients who receive rehabilitation services only after developing significant disability. Rarely are they adequately screened for emerging impairments that could be remediated at early stages. Many functional assessment tools that have been validated in non cancer illnesses or the elderly effectively discriminate levels of functioning in advanced cancer patients (Cheville, 2005).

Rehabilitation medicine professionals often have limited exposure to cancer patients during their training. Lack of familiarity with cancer-related impairments limits caregivers' willingness to deliver established and effective modalities to cancer patients. For many rehabilitation specialists, the trajectory of functional decline in cancer is difficult to predict since it deviates from that seen in other major rehabilitative diagnoses (Gillis, 2003). This can lead to a delay or failure in the delivery of appropriate interventions at effective intensities. Conversely, rehabilitation professionals unfamiliar with cancer prognoses may endorse inappropriately aggressive and costly therapies.

Primary care providers, oncologists and palliative medicine providers may have limited diagnostic acumen for cancer-related neuro- and musculoskeletal pathology; they may have limited capacity to detect biomechanical abnormalities given the absence of rehabilitation exposure in most medical school curricula. Few clinicians have observed an integrated, interdisciplinary rehabilitation service at any point in their professional experience. Oncologists may focus only on curative interventions in response to the treatment agenda of their patients. Patients may conceal subtle deficits for fear that their oncologist may defer, interrupt or discontinue a potentially curative treatment. Alternatively, patients may fear that these symptoms are harbingers of disease progression. Many patients lack access to education on how to identify and address evolving impairments.

Reimbursement barriers limit the patients' access to rehabilitation providers. The federal Balanced Budget Act has diminished access for patients to rehabilitative services in skilled nursing facilities following hospitalizations. The reduced lengths of acute hospitalization diminish access to hospital-based physical, occupational, and speech therapists. Reduced length of stay also limits the ability of rehabilitation professionals to monitor the effectiveness of specific interventions and modify them accordingly. Ironically, while payers may reimburse expensive, new anti-neoplastic modalities that are of marginal benefit access, to established rehabilitative interventions such as joint injections may be precluded due to capitation of services. Many physical medicine physicians may find nerve conduction studies and interventional analgesic approaches to be more financially sustaining than the non- interventional approaches emphasized in cancer rehabilitation which are cognitively demanding and therefore time consuming for providers.

11. Conclusion

The prevalence of cancer-related disability can be expected to grow as the number of patients living with a history of cancer increases. Cancer rehabilitation offers the opportunity to preserve function and enhance quality of life. Rehabilitative goals potentate patients' dignity, self image, and social integration. Rehabilitation professionals familiar with cancer patients' frailty can effectively preserve functional integrity in tandem with efforts to eradicate the underlying disease. Lack of cancer-specific expertise among physiatrists, notably understanding of malignant disease trajectories, risks of treatment toxicities, and current cancer therapies remains a barrier to successful rehabilitation. In order to improve cancer patients' access to effective care it is critical that cancer-related expertise be cultivated among rehabilitation specialists and that these professionals be integrated into disease management systems. This may lessen the medical and economic burden of cancer.

Glossary

Neuropathy: An abnormality of peripheral nerves related to infection, inflammation, medication use, metabolic causes and malignancy.

Plexopathy: injury to either the brachial plexus or lumbosacral plexus. The brachial plexus is a collection of nerves that arises from the cervical and upper thoracic nerve roots. The lumbosacral plexus arises from the nerve roots that emerge from the lumbosacral spine

Myopathy: An impairment in the activity of muscles which may be related to inflammation, endocrine, malignant, infectious or metabolic causes

Lymphedema: swelling or edema of an extremity that can be caused by malignant or surgical disruption of lymphatic structures.

Pleura: epithelial lining of the inner aspect of the thorax and outer surface of the lung.

Sarcoma: solid organ malignant tumor which can occur in bone, cartilage and muscle.

Proprioreception: The sensation of vibration or joint position.

Anasarca: Generalized body swelling that occurs in advanced multisystems organ failure and congestive heart failure.

Leukopenia: An abnormally low white blood cell count

Thrombocytopenia: An abnormally low platelet count

PCA pump: A patient-controlled analgesic device which enables the patient to self-administer analgesic (pain controlling) medications. These pumps can be connected to epidural or venous access ports and can be used for long-term pain management in patients with life-limiting conditions.

References

Aaronson, N.K. Ahmedzai, S., Bergman, B., Bullinger, M., Cull, A., Duez, N.J., Filiberti, H. Fleshner, H., Fleischmann, S.B., and DeHaes, J.C. (1993). The European Organization for Research and Treatment of Cancer QLQ-C30: a quality-of-life instrument for use in international clinical trials in oncology. *Journal of the National Cancer Institute.* 85(5):365-376.

Anderson, F., Downing, G.M., Hill, J., Casorso, L., and Lerch, N. (1996). Palliative Performance Scale (PPS): a new tool. *Journal of Palliative Care.* 12(1):5-11.

Breitbart, W., Rosenfeld, B., Pessin, H., Kaim, M., Funesti-Esch, J., Galietta, M., Nelson, C.J., and Brescia, R. (2000). Depression, hopelessness, and desire for hastened death in terminally ill patients with cancer. *JAMA.* 284(22):2907-2911.

Buccheri, G., Ferrigno, D., and Tamburini, M. (1996). Karnofsky and ECOG performance status scoring in lung cancer: a prospective, longitudinal study of 536 patients from a single institution. *European Journal of Cancer.* 32(A):1135-1141.

Byock, I.R. and Merriman, M.P. (1998). Measuring quality of life for patients with terminal illness: The Missoula-VITAS quality of life index. *Palliative Medicine.* 12, 231-244.

Cella, D.F., Bonomi, A.E., Hahn, E.A., Bjordal, K., Sperner-Unterweger, B., Gangeri, L., Bergman, B., Willems-Groot, J., Hanquet, P., and Zittoun, R. (1996). Multilingual translation of the functional assessment of Cancer Therapy (FACT) quality of life measurement system. *Quality of Life Research.* 5(3):309-320.

Chang, V.T., Hwang, S.S., Feuerman, M.F., Kasimis, B.S., and Thaler, H.T. (2000). The Memorial Symptom Assessment Scale Short form (MSAS-SF) *Cancer.* 89(5): 1162-1171.

Cheville, A., and Kornblith, A.: Impairment–associated distress in stage IV breast cancer. Presented at the 63rd Annual Assembly of Rehabilitation Medicine, Orlando, Fl, November 21-24, 2002.

Cheville, A. (2005). Cancer Rehabilitation. *Seminars in Oncology.* 32(2):219-224.

Cleeland, C.S., and Ryan, K.M. (1994). Pain Assessment: global use of the Brief Pain Inventory. *Annals of the Academy of Medicine of Singapore.* 23:129-138.

Coleman, E.A., Hall-Barrow, J., Coon, S., and Stewart, C.B. (2003). Facilitating exercise adherence for patients with multiple myeloma. *Clinical Journal Oncology Nursing.* 7(5):529-34, 40.

Dietz, J.J. (1974). Rehabilitation of the cancer patient: It's role in the scheme of comprehensive care. *Clinical Bulletin.* 4:104-107.

Dietz, J.H. Jr. (1980). Adaptive rehabilitation in cancer *Current Problems in Cancer.* 1980 5(5):1-56.

Dimeo, F.C., Tilman, M.H., Bertz H, Kanz, L., Mertelsmann, R., and Keul, J. (1997). Aerobic exercise in the rehabilitation of cancer patients after high dose chemotherapy and autologous peripheral stem cell transplantation. *Cancer.* 79 (9):1717-1722.

Endicott, J. (1983). Measurement of depression in patients with cancer. *Cancer.* 53: 2243-2248.

Friendenreich, C.M. and Courneya, K.S. (1996). Exercise as rehabilitation for cancer patients. *Clinical Journal of Sports Medicine.* 6(4):237-244.

Garman, K.S., McConnell, E.S., and Cohen, H.J. (2004). Inpatient care for elderly cancer patients: the role of geriatric evalution and management Units in fulfilling goals of care. *Critical Reviews in Oncology/Hematology.* 51(3):241-247.

Gillis, T.A. 2003. Rehabilitation medicine interventions. In: Breura E.D, and Portenoy, R.K. (eds.), *Cancer Pain: Assessment and Management,* Cambridge University Press, New York, NY, pp. 238-260.

Granger, C.V., Albrecht, G.L., and Hamilton, B.B. (1979). Outcome of comprehensive medical rehabilitation: Measurement by PULSES and the Barthel Index. *Arch Phys Med Rehabil.* 60(4):145-154.

Hamilton, B.B., Granger, C.V., Sherwin, F.S. et al. A uniform national data system for medical rehabilitation. In: Fuhrer M.J. (ed.). *Rehabilitation Outcomes: Analysis and Measurement.* Brooks Publishing Co. Baltimore, 1987, 137.

Harvey, R., Jellinek, H., and Habeck, R. Cancer Rehabilitation. (1982). An analysis of 36 program approaches. *Journal of the American Medical Association.* 247(15):2127-2131.

Hearn, J., and Higginson, I.J. (1999). Development and validation of a core outcome measure for palliative care: the palliative care outcome scale. *Quality & Health Care.* 8:219-227.

Hillel, A. and Patten, C. (1990). Neck dissection: Morbidity and rehabilitation. *Cancer Treatment and Research.* 52:133-147.

Kaasa, T., and Wessel, J. (2001). The Edmonton Functional Assessment Tool: Further development and validation for use in palliative care. *Journal of Palliative Care.* 17(1):5-11.

Karnell, L., Funk, G., and Hoffman, H. (2000). Assessing head and neck cancer patient outcome domains. *Head and Neck.* 22:6-11.

Karnofsky, D.A., and Burchenal, J.H. (1949). The clinical evaluation of chemotherapeutic agents in cancer. In: McLeod CM Ed. *Evaluation of Chemotherapeutic Agents.* Columbia University Press, New York, pp. 191-205.

King, J.C., Williams, R.P., and McAnelly, R.D. (1994). Rehabilitation of tumor amputees and limb salvage patients. *Phys Med Rehabil State Art Rev.* 8:297-319.

Ko, D., Lerner, R., Klose, G., and Cosimi, A.B. (1998). Effective treatment of lymphedema in the extremities. *Archives of Surgery.* 133(4):452-458.

Larto, M. A randomized trial comparing radiation therapy alone with chemotherapy for squamous cell cancer of the head and neck (SCHNC): Quality of life (QoL) assessment. *Proceedings of the American Society of Clinical Oncology.* 17, 382a (Abstract # 1460).

Lehman, J., De Lisa, J., and Warren, C. (1978). Cancer Rehabilitation: Assessment of need, development, and evaluation of a model of care. *Archives of Physical Medicine and Rehabilitation.* 59:410-419.

Loge, J.H., and Kaasa, S. (1998). Fatigue and cancer-prevalence, correlates and measurement. *Progress in Palliative Care.* 6:43-47.

Loprinzi, C.L., Laurie, J.A., Wieand, H.S., Krook, J.E., Novotny, P.J., Kugler, J.W., Bartel, J., Law, M., Bateman, M., and Klatt, N.E. (1994). Prospective evaluation of prognostic variables from patient completed questionnaires. *Journal of Clinical Oncology.* 12(3):601-607.

Lynn, J. and Adamson, D. (2003). Rand Corporation Living well at the end of life: adapting healthcare to serious chronic illness in old age. White paper. Washington D: RAND Corporation. Available online at www.rand.org/publications/WP/WP137.

Mahoney, F.L. and Barthel, D.W. (1965). Functional evaluation: The Barthel Index. *Maryland State Medical Journal.* 14:61.

Marciniak, C.M., Silwa, J.A., Spill G., Heinemann, A.W., and Semik, P.E. (1996). Functional outcomes following rehabilitayion of the cancer patient. *Archives of Physical Medicine and Rehabilitation.* 77(1):54-57.

Mcilvoy, L., Spain, D.A., Raque, G., Vitaz, T., Boaz, P., and Meyer, K. (2001). Successful incorporation of the severe head injury guidelines into a phased-outcome clinical pathway. *Journal of Neuroscience Nursing.* 33(2):72-78, 82.

Mellette, S. Development and utilization of rehabilitation and continuing care resources for cancer patients. (Final report, June 1974 to July 1977) Contract N01-CN-65287. Richmond, VA, Medical College of Virginia/Virginia Commonwealth University Cancer Center, 1977.

Mor, V., Laliberte, L., Morris, J.N., and Wiemann, M. (1984). The Karnofsky Performance Status Scale. An examination of its reliability and validity in a research setting. *Cancer.* 53(9):2002-2007.

Natterlund, B., Gunnarsson, L.G., and Ahlstrom, G. (2000). Disability, coping and quality of life in individuals with muscular dystrophy: a prospective study over five years. *Disability and Rehabilitation.* 22(17):776-785.

O'Brien, K., Nixon, S., Tynan, A.M., and Glazier, R.H. (2004(a)). Effectiveness of aerobic exercise in adults living with HIV/AIDS:Systematic Review. *Medicine and Science in Sports Exerc.* 36(10):1659-1666.

O'Brien, K., Nixon, S., Glazier, R.H., and Tynan, A.M. (2004(b)). Progressive resistive exercises for adults living with HIV/AIDS. *Cochrane Database Syst Rev.* (4) CD004248

Oldervall, L.M., Kaasa, S., Hjermstad, M.J., Lund, J.A., and Loge, J.H. (2004) Physical exercise results in the subjective well-being of a few or is effective rehabilitation treatment for all cancer patients. *European Journal of Cancer.* 40(7):951-962.

O'Mahony, S., Kornblith, A., Goulet, J., Abbatiello, G., Clarke, B., Kless-Siegel, S., Breitbart, W., and Payne, R. (2005). Desire for hastened death, cancer pain and depression: report of a longitudinal observational study. *Journal of Pain and Symptom Management.* 29(5):446-457.

O'Mahony, S., Blank, A.E., Zallman, L., and Selwyn, P.A. (2005). The Benefits of a hospital-based inpatient palliative care consultation service: preliminary outcome data. *Journal of Palliative Medicine.* 8(5):1033-1041.

Pickett, M., Mock, V., Ropka, M.E., Cameron, L., Coleman, M., and Podewils L. (2002). Adherance to moderate intensity exercise during breast cancer treatment. *Cancer Practice.* 10(6):284-292.

Spielberger, C.D. (1983). *Manual for the State-Trait Anxiety Inventory (STAI).* Consulting Psychologists Press, Palo Alto, CA.

Teichmann, J.V. (2002). Oncological rehabilitation: evaluation of the efficiency of inpatient rehabilitation. *Rehabilitation* (Stutt) 41(1):53-62.

Tiep, BL. (1997). Disease management of COPD with pulmonary rehabilitation. *Chest.* 112(6):1630-1656.

Terrell, J., Fisher, S., and Wolf, G. (1998). Long term quality of life after treatment of laryngeal cancer. *Archives of Otolaryngology-Head and Neck Surgery.* 124:964-971.

Waldron, D., O'Boyle, C.A., Kearney, M., Moriarty, M., and Carney, D. (1999). Quality-of-life measurement in advanced cancer: assessing the individual. *Journal of Clinical Oncology.* 17:3603-3611.

Weymuller, E.A., Yueh, B., Deleyiannis, F.W., Kuntz, A.L., Alsarraf, R., and Coltrer M.D. (2000). Quality of life in patients with head and neck cancer: lessons learned from 549 prospectively evaluated patients. *Archives of Otolaryngology–Head and Neck Surgery.* 126(3):329-335.

Willems, D.L., Daniels, E.R., van der Wal, G., van der Maas, P.J., Emanuel, E.J. (2000). Attitudes and practices concerning the end of life: a comparison between physicians from the United States and from The Netherlands. *Archives of Internal Medicine.* 160(1):63-68.

Winningham, M.L., Nail, L., Barton-Burke, M, Brophy, L., Cimprich, B., Jones, L.S., Pickard-Holley, S., Rhodes, V., St Pierre, B., and Beck, S. (1994). Fatigue and the cancer experience: the state of the knowledge. *Oncology Nursing Forum.* 21:23-36.

Yates, J.W., Chalmer, B., and McKegney, P. (1980). Evaluation of patients with advanced cancer using the Karnofsky Performance Status scale. *Cancer.* 45(8):2220-2224.

Yoshioka, H.: Rehabilitation for terminal cancer patients. (1994). *American Journal of Physical Medicine and Rehabilitation.* 73:199-206.

Zigmond, A.S. and Snaith, R.P. (1983). The Hospital Anxiety and Depression Scale. *Acta Psychiatrica Scandinavica.* 67:361-370.

6
HIV/AIDS and Palliative Care: Models of Care and Policy Issues

Peter A. Selwyn MD MPH, Linda Robinson PhD,
Martha G. Dale MPH, and Ruth McCorkle PhD FAAN

1. Introduction

The past two decades have seen both the emergence of AIDS as a new, life-threatening illness and its conversion from a rapidly fatal to a manageable chronic disease. This pattern has been most marked in industrialized countries where the promise of HIV-specific therapies has been realized for many individuals living with HIV. However, even in the era of 'highly active antiretroviral therapy' (HAART), AIDS remains an important cause of morbidity and mortality in many young adult populations, and attention to chronic disease and palliative care issues remains an essential aspect of clinical care and program planning.

In the early 1980's, AIDS quickly became the leading cause of death for young adults in the United States (CDC, 1991). With advances in AIDS care and HIV-specific therapy, mortality rates began to decline in the mid-1990's, and accelerated with the introduction of the protease inhibitors in 1996 (CDC, 1997; Palella *et al.*, 1998; CDC, 2000; Wong *et al.*, 2000; Chiasson *et al.*, 1999; Egger *et al.*, 1997). However, the decline in death rates has since plateaued, and there remain approximately 15,000 deaths per year from HIV/AIDS (CDC, 2000). Moreover, the declines in death rates have not been uniform across all populations affected by HIV/AIDS, and decreasing mortality has not been as pronounced among African-Americans and Latinos as it has been among whites (CDC, 2000, 2001). Moreover, recent surveillance data and clinical studies have indicated that mortality

PETER A. SELWYN • Professor and Chairman, Department of Family and Social Medicine, Montefiore Medical Center, Albert Einstein College of Medicine, 3544 Jerome Avenue, Bronx, NY 10467.   LINDA ROBINSON • Associate Professor, University of San Diego, Hahn School of Nursing and Health Science, 5998 Alcala Park, San Diego, CA 92110-2492.   MARTHA G. DALE • Executive Director, Leeway, Inc, 40 Albert St., New Haven, CT 06511.   RUTH McCORKLE • The Florence S. Wald Professor of Nursing, Director, Center for Excellence in Chronic Illness Care, Yale University School of Nursing, 100 Church Street South, PO Box 9740, New Haven, CT. 06536-0740.

among patients with HIV has been steadily increasing from common co-morbidities such as hepatitis B and C, co-occurring malignancies (both AIDS-defining and non-AIDS-defining cancers), and substance abuse-related deaths (Sansone and Frengly, 2000; Selwyn *et al.*, 2000; Puoti *et al.*, 2001; www.cdc.gov, 2001; Kravcik *et al.*, 1997; Valdez *et al.*, 2001). In addition, for certain patients, even the benefit of HAART is not always attainable, due to lack of access to care, inability to adhere to effective treatment regimens, active substance use or other psychiatric illness, progressive viral resistance despite therapy, serious other co-morbidities, or unmanageable drug toxicities. Moreover, the incidence of new HIV infections in the United States is not believed to have decreased, and has remained stable at approximately 40,000 new cases per year (CDC, 2001). As a result of these trends, AIDS-related mortality continues to be an important phenomenon, even while the number of patients living with HIV (i.e., the prevalence of AIDS) has actually increased (Figure 6.1) (CDC, 2000, 2001).

In the pre-HAART era, AIDS was a uniformly fatal, relentlessly progressive illness, characterized by multiple opportunistic infections, swift decline, and death within months of diagnosis. The impact of disease-specific treatment on the natural history of HIV infection has now resulted in a much more variable trajectory of illness for many patients. For some, HAART has meant the possibility of full return of function and health, while for others, treatment has meant the 'conversion of death to disability,' with the emergence of a chronic

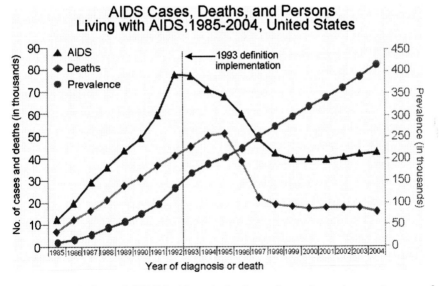

FIGURE 6.1. Estimated AIDS incidence*, deaths, and prevalence, by quarter-year of diagnosis/death—United States, 1985–2004
*Adjust for reporting delays.

disease phase characterized by exacerbations, remissions, and eventual death (Selwyn *et al.*, 2000) as the survival time from diagnosis to death has lengthened (Lee *et al.*, 2001). Over a remarkably short period of time, the historical evolution of HIV disease – for which the stereotypic disease course from diagnosis to death first resembled that of certain predominantly fatal cancers (e.g., pancreas, lung) – has shifted to a trajectory more typical of chronic, progressive illnesses (e.g., congestive heart failure, chronic obstructive pulmonary disease, hepatic cirrhosis), with much more variability in outcomes (Figure 6.2) (Lynn, 1997).

In this context, the management of AIDS as a chronic disease has had increasingly important implications for the organization and delivery of clinical services, and has required the development of new models of care to respond to the emerging needs of a population along the continuum of long-term care. Notwithstanding the dramatic therapeutic advances in HAART, it is important to recognize that the curative vs. palliative dichotomy in HIV care is a false one. The need to incorporate both palliative and curative approaches in HIV care may indeed be more important than it was in the pre-HAART era: the potential availability of effective treatment does not give clinicians the luxury of ignoring the important issues posed by a chronic progressive illness and its management over time (Selwyn and Arnold, 1998). On a programmatic level, the availability and effectiveness of HAART does not obviate the need to develop systems of care for those patients who are further along the continuum of progressive, incurable illness, and who may have complex and overlapping medical, psychiatric, and social needs.

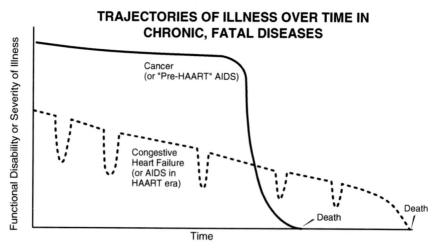

FIGURE 6.2. Trajectories of illness over time in chronic, fatal diseases

AIDS has always presented unique psychosocial problems for patients, families, and care providers: a life-threatening illness affecting young adults, often with multiple infected family members, raising difficult issues of premature death, unfinished business, legacy, and survivorship. The association between AIDS, poverty, and racial-ethnic minority populations in the United States further compounds the vulnerability of many patients living with HIV/AIDS, and there remains a significant degree of stigma, fear, and prejudice regarding AIDS within the society as a whole. It is critical for decisions regarding planning for chronic disease management and palliative care to address issues concerning perceived withdrawal of care (or perceived 'second-class' or less-than-aggressive care), cultural differences regarding advance care preferences, and the marginalization of vulnerable populations (Mouton *et al.*, 1997; Wenger *et al.*, 2001).

This chapter addresses issues and models of care relevant to health services development and planning for HIV/AIDS as a chronic disease, including the continuum of care from outpatient, home-based, to skilled nursing facility and other institutional settings.

2. Models of Care for HIV/AIDS as a Chronic Disease

Health care services for people with HIV/AIDS have been guided by various models for over two decades. What lessons have been learned regarding the effectiveness of variant models for providing such complex and ever-changing care?

2.1. Case Management

The most predominant model of care described in the literature has been a case management model, as living with HIV/AIDS requires ongoing coordination of medical care and social services. Case managers provide disease-specific knowledge required to manage the HIV/AIDS illness course, access federal and state entitlements as well as community level services, and obtain specialized services for patients with co-morbidities such as mental illness and substance abuse. While arranging these services would be complex for anyone, HIV/AIDS disproportionately affects vulnerable populations who are perhaps least able to coordinate their care. Through coordination of services, case management can successfully maximize community based care, thus saving health care dollars by avoiding costly inpatient care (Mitchell and Anderson, 2000).

How case management is defined across health care settings can range from coordination of services to providing direct patient care. In an analysis of the tasks and activities of HIV/AIDS case managers in the tri-county region of New York State in 1998, Grube and Chernesky (2001) categorized case managers' tasks and activities into three core areas: disease management, entitlements/benefits, and essential services. Half of the actions reported addressed disease management (doctors, medications,

AIDS information, etc), 45% addressed securing essential services (clothing, housing, transportation, etc) and 5% involved accessing entitlements (Medicaid, public assistance, SSI, etc). Despite the lively debate surrounding what discipline is best prepared to case manage patients with HIV infection, it appears from the activities that case managers routinely carry out, no one discipline is prepared to case manage the wide array of service needs required. Multidisciplinary case management services would provide the ideal preparation for this model of care with illness specialty trained case managers arranging for the bulk of services that have been shown to be required.

In an effort to move beyond *process* evaluation and examine *outcomes* of case management programs for people with HIV/AIDS, Lehrman, *et al.* (2001) reported nearly 7,050 service needs among 588 patients recruited from 28 different agencies. Women, patients with children living with them, the inadequately housed and patients without a high school diploma were found to have the most needs. Services directly provided for by the case management agency were arranged for and utilized more frequently than services that had to be referred to an outside agency. Based on these findings the authors concluded that case management models that provide intensive services to women with children and house multiple services in addition to case management within a single agency provide a more ideal model of care. Providing different levels of case management service to different populations requires flexibility in how resources are distributed.

2.2. Integrated Care Models

The idea of housing multiple services under one roof or providing a "one-stop-shopping" model of care is not new and is an efficient model of care for chronically ill populations. Since the development of HAART, HIV care has become highly specialized and complex. Effective viral suppression is dependent on practitioners who are knowledgeable about state of the science therapeutic modalities. Yet patients need care that attends to all of their problems; those related and unrelated to their HIV infection. Vulnerable populations such as the mentally ill and those with substance use issues have difficulty accessing care when it requires dealing with multiple, fragmented health care systems. Further, HIV remains a highly stigmatizing condition and having to "come out" to multiple providers about one's sexual, drug, and social history presents a barrier to receiving care for the most needy and hard-to-reach HIV infected populations. Models of care that specialize in HIV care but refer other services elsewhere are less than ideal.

One example of an integrated care model that has been highly successful is the Fenway Community Health Model which began as a neighborhood clinic in Boston in 1971 and grew in response to the AIDS epidemic (Mayer *et al.*, 2001). The Fenway Program's offerings are broad, including primary medical care and HIV specialty care, obstetrics, gynecology, gerontology, podiatry, dermatology services, mental health and addiction services, and a wide array of complementary therapies. Besides providing the broad array of needed services, this model's success has also been attributed to a focus on cultural competence. The Fenway Community Health Model is identified as 1 of only 9 lesbian, gay, bisexual and transgendered (LGBT) community health centers in the United States. In addition to direct patient care services, Fenway has developed programs to combat homophobic violence, provides community education about LGBT issues and education of health providers about LGBT issues and reproductive planning services that include artificial insemination. Ineffective patient-provider communication has been shown to contribute to social disparities in health care (Cooper and Roter, 2003). Providing care, as Fenway has, to patients with sensitivity and commitment to their unique cultural issues may be one of the key attributes of an ideal model of HIV care.

Another successful model for providing integrated care, outside of housing services under one roof, is the Personalized Nursing Light Model (Anderson *et al.*, 2003). The process of care guided by this model focuses on locating hard-to-reach patients that have been lost to follow-up, linking them to health care services, and integrating care among different providers. The central tenet of the model is that when patients are linked one-on-one to a nurse, they can more readily achieve positive health outcomes. Nurses accompany patients to their health care appointments and mutually set goals with patients for improving well-being. The effectiveness of the model has been supported in several studies where patients receiving this model of care showed declines in substance use, declines in depression and psychological distress and improvements in global well being (Anderson *et al.*, 2003; Anderson and Hockman, 1997). Providing care using this model is labor resource intensive in an era of extreme nursing shortages. Yet, for certain populations, HIV infected substance abusers in particular, a model such as this may be necessary as traditional case management models have not proven successful (Sorensen *et al.*, 2003).

2.3. Palliative Care and End-of-Life Issues

If models of HIV care are to be effective, they must address patient needs across the entire illness trajectory and be transferable across care settings in order to provide seamless care. When patients with HIV become increasingly symptomatic, the issue of curative versus palliative models of care must be considered. The HIV/AIDS illness trajectory challenges the traditional approach of viewing curative and palliative care models as mutually exclusive (Foley *et al.*, 1995). As noted above, the HIV/AIDS trajectory in the HAART era does not follow a linear, inevitable progression to death. Functional declines do not occur in uniform patterns, and patients' abilities to care for themselves frequently change (Fleishman and Crystal, 1998). Advanced therapeutics have revived patients on the verge of dying and returned them to a more stable illness phase. For this reason, symptomatic patients with HIV/AIDS eligible for hospice services to relieve their suffering have often been reluctant to accept hospice care as doing so might mean having to forego curative care.

In order to provide better options for patients with HIV/AIDS who are symptomatic and declining in their self care ability, home-based models of care have been developed to provide both curative and palliative care. The Visiting Nurse Association of Los Angeles and San Diego Palliative Home Healthcare provide good exemplars for blending curative and palliative care paradigms (Cherin et al., 1998; Oppenheim et al., 2002). In both settings interdisciplinary health care professionals provide curative and palliative services. Nurse case managers provide direct care and work with social workers to coordinate care between hospital admissions, clinic appointments, and other care providers. Both models provide extensive clinical training to their staff in curative and palliative HIV/AIDS care modalities and conduct regular care conferences with a physician.

Whether combining the care paradigms could be cost effective was of concern as health care expenditures at the end of life remain the highest in our health care system (Cherin et al., 1998). To examine this, data were collected from 549 AIDS patients admitted for home care services at the Visiting Nurse Association of Los Angeles (Cherin et al., 1998). On admission to home care patients were randomly assigned to either a traditional home care model or a model blending curative and palliative care. An eight percent reduction in service delivery costs were found with the blended home care model compared with the traditional home care model supporting the cost effectiveness of this approach. Increasingly, these types of models –able to provide both disease-specific, 'curative' therapies and expert palliative and end-of-life care – will be needed to meet the complex clinical challenges of HIV/AIDS in the HAART era.

The preceding overview has focused on existing models for providing community-based, outpatient HIV/AIDS care, developed to improve patient outcomes and control health care costs. While no singular model of care has addressed all needs of patients with HIV/AIDS, incorporating these critical elements will help address the disparities currently seen in delivering HIV/AIDS care. HIV/AIDS care is so complex and broad, spanning medical and social aspects of care, that incorporating a multi-disciplinary approach is essential, focused on specific sub-populations which differ by gender, ethnicity, disease stage, and HIV risk category. Special efforts need to be made to assist vulnerable HIV/AIDS patients to access care whether the model of care integrates services under one roof or facilitates access across multiple locations.

2.4. Post-Acute Long Term Care in Institutional Settings

The early days of the HIV/AIDS epidemic, when patients were living long enough to need ongoing care services but not necessarily in an acute health care setting, presented a care delivery problem for communities. Challenged with limited alternatives, a number of communities decided that the best alternative to relieve the hospital census pressure was to develop alternative care settings. These typically urban communities, with a sufficient population base and state legislatures willing to write new reimbursement methodologies or public health code licensing regulations, addressed these health care delivery needs by developing primarily skilled nursing facilities that would be able to provide sub-acute nursing services for patients with HIV/AIDS at a lesser cost then acute care hospitals. (AIDS Housing of Washington, 2003, Silha)

Changes in the epidemic since the mid-1990's have led to programmatic and organizational implications for the facilities that were earlier developed as an alternative to acute-care settings. Notwithstanding the dramatic benefits of HAART, co-morbidities such as addiction, co-existing medical conditions, and psychological disorders all complicate the chronic care of patients with HIV/AIDS (Columbia University, 2000; Greenberg et al., 2000; Corless and Nicholas, 2000). The coexistence of HIV infection with substance abuse, mental illness, homelessness and/or other social factors has resulted in a population of patients who are particularly susceptible to medication non-adherence, medication toxicity and inaccessibility to health services (Selwyn, 1996; Bangsburg et al., 1997; Moore et al., 1994). These multiply diagnosed patients incur higher treatment costs than other persons living with HIV/AIDS (Greenberg et al., 2000), and require enhanced long-term disease management practices.

Additionally, for some of these clients, their stays in skilled nursing facilities (SNF's) are extended because of limited post-SNF discharge alternatives to care for the combined needs of HIV/AIDS, the co-morbidities of substance abuse, chronic medical disease, mental illness, and a lack of stable housing and family environments. Because multiply-diagnosed patients have difficulty engaging in and adhering to their prescribed treatment regimes, the likelihood exists that these individuals will receive care outside of an institutional setting is low. The lack of a continuum of care that will ensure long-term multiple disease management after discharge from an institutional setting increases the chance that the individual's condition will deteriorate again, resulting in readmission to either a hospital or the skilled nursing facility (Gomez, 2004).

Pressure to return to community living is strong among this generally young population – institutional living is not a preferred choice in clients who, now relieved of the prospect of imminent death, expect to rebuild their lives as they once had envisioned for themselves. Comprehensive and seamless medical, social and residential programs specifically targeted to the most vulnerable of the HIV/AIDS population have been slow to develop in response to the emergence of the chronic disease phase of the epidemic and the lack of such programs and, ultimately delays discharges from SNFs for many of these clients (Goulet et al., 2000). Experience among providers has proven that quite often it is either the substance abuse and/or mental health diagnoses, in addition to loneliness and placement in a neighborhood with a high prevalence of substance abuse, that can lead to medication non-adherence and readmission to the cycle of illness, hospitalization and discharge to post-acute long term settings (Chorost, 2003). SNF care teams become increasingly reticent to seek discharge options for these clients and instead "protect" these clients by encouraging that they stay in the skilled nursing facility. Additionally, because a large proportion of the multiply diagnosed HIV infected persons may also be homeless or in imminent danger of homelessness or are indigent (De Mello, 2000), there are few residential alternatives to the SNF. A study at Leeway, Inc., an HIV/AIDS dedicated SNF in New Haven, CT, found that although there were not significant differences in reported reasons for admission to the SNF, patients admitted with co-morbid disorders had more favorable functional characteristics and lower death rates than those without co-morbidities. The authors suggest that the individuals with other co-morbidities were often at a less advanced stage of their HIV illness and should have been discharged sooner (Goulet et al., 2000).

We are now witnessing a repeat of the care-delivery dilemma that is credited with the creation of AIDS specific SNFs, although this time occurring further along the care continuum. What was experienced in the first instance was the need to create specialized skilled nursing facilities for the purposes of relieving the strain on hospital-level care. Now, we are finding that as the impact of the disease has changed, in large part due to the intervention of new drug therapies, SNFs are likewise experiencing the same phenomenon they were intended to alleviate. In a word, the skilled nursing facilities for HIV/AIDS patients have become the victims of their own success.

How is the health care administrator to respond when confronted by the need to insure that necessary beds are available for those most in need as well as the responsibility to be able to successfully and responsibly discharge those with a potential for community living and finally, the need to create service components to support successful discharge planning? The following section will address these issues both thematically and with reference to the experience of Leeway, the freestanding AIDS-dedicated long-term care facility in New Haven, CT (Goulet et al., 2000; Selwyn et al., 2000).

2.5. The Current Challenge for Institutional Long Term Care Providers

There will continue to exist a tension between community living and institutional care for the client with a complex, chronic disease or disability. The intent should be to always strive to find the highest optimum level of independent living for the client in the least restrictive environment. As a necessary prerequisite to building new care alternatives in the community setting, it will always be the long term care administrator's responsibility to design and secure funding sources for enhanced medical and behavioral health care programs *within* the SNF to bring clients to a level of independent living capacity *before* considering discharge to the community. The provision of life skills training, substance abuse counseling, and individual and group psychiatric treatment are examples of unique services required for this population to maximize success after SNF discharge and ultimately ensure ongoing medication adherence for HIV/AIDS. However, these are programs not typically reimbursed in the long-term care institutional setting by conventional Medicaid or Medicare programs. Seeking federal, state and private grant funds to pay for these programs has been a strategy to bring these services into the nursing home and better prepare clients for discharge.

Agencies such as the United Way, the federal Housing and Urban Development Agency and their Housing Opportunities for Persons With AIDS (HOPWA), and state Medicaid, mental health and/or addiction services agencies are examples of sources that have been successfully used in some initiatives to cover the costs of alternative programming that is directly targeted at the treatment of substance abuse, mental illness and co-occurring social problems in long term care facilities serving patients with HIV/AIDS.

One may be tempted to ask if there is now or will be in the future a need to create more nursing home beds for the HIV/AIDS population. Despite the fact that the number of persons living with HIV/AIDS will continue to grow, it is unlikely that state governments will endorse the addition of new dedicated-long term care facilities. The flurry of new AIDS-dedicated skilled nursing homes that came on line in the early to mid-1990's will most likely not be replicated as states experience growing Medicaid program expenditures. It is not that the capital costs for dedicated SNF AIDS beds are significantly greater that the average geriatric long term facility, but rather the per diem cost of care, which would include the increased staffing levels, medication costs and medical supply costs. The average cost of a Medicaid AIDS-dedicated bed per diem can be as much as two times the cost of a typical geriatric Medicaid reimbursement per diem rate. From a health policy perspective, the presence of additional nursing home beds may relieve the natural pressure to seek less institutionalized and less costly community-based settings that promote a better quality of life.

The best solution then is to make more efficient use of the current complement of beds and at the same time advocate for a broader array of support and residential services in the community that provide a safe, alternative care choice. Accelerating the "through-put" of HIV/AIDS nursing home residents back to the community and freeing up beds for those with more complex medical needs is the best solution for payers and patients alike.

Typically, disability advocacy groups have led the effort to define new care delivery methods when existing services do not maximize the independence of the client. This has been true for the developmentally disabled population, physically disabled, the traumatic brain injury population and for the frail elderl (Reester et al., 2004). In each case, there have been landmark legislative initiatives in states to de-institutionalize these populations with the intent of providing care in the least restrictive environment while enhancing self-direction and quality of life.

Using special legislative initiatives for a specific disabled population, Medicaid waivers can provide financing for community supports as an alternative to institutional care. Section 1915(c) of the Social Security Act allows states to apply for waivers to provide home and community-based services as an alternative to institutional care in a hospital, nursing home, or intermediate care facility. If approved, these waivers allow states to target specific populations and determine the long-term care services they wish to offer and do so in a manner that caters to the specific needs of a specific target population (www.cms.hhs.gov). Unfortunately, unless the legislation is broadly written to capture a wide range of disability groups, these alternative financing arrangements typically are not accessible by others sharing similar long term care institutional constraints but with different diagnoses.

Medicaid funding for a comprehensive array of home and community-based services for persons with HIV/AIDS has only been secured for 14 states (Oderna *et al.*, 2005). However, when a Medicaid claims data analysis was conducted in 2002 on the potential cost-savings benefits of such a waiver program for persons in Connecticut who are Medicaid participants and who currently reside in skilled nursing facilities, a potential savings of $1.4 million was projected for the first two years of the program and $4 million for five years (Gomez, 2004). The administrative staff at the Leeway skilled nursing facility in New Haven, Connecticut had requested assistance from the Yale School of Epidemiology and Public Health with this research in order to provide cost-savings data that would provide a convincing economic argument for such a waiver in Connecticut. Work continues at the both the state legislature and among state agency administrators to prepare an application for such a waiver to pay for intensive case management services for the state's chronically ill population with HIV/AIDS, along with a wide array of support services such as transportation, home-delivered meals and homemaker services, to name a few.

Through a partnership with other non-profit organizations in the local community, Leeway has developed specialized, scattered site and clustered supportive housing units into which its most vulnerable clients can be discharged. The Corporation for Supportive Housing, a national non-profit organization dedicated to ending homelessness, brought together agencies like Leeway and non-profit housing developers to secure funding for supportive housing units for those who are homeless or at risk of homelessness and who have psychiatric disabilities or chemical dependency or both (documents.csh.org, 2004). The Connecticut Supportive Housing Pilots Initiative helped agency collaboratives secured funding for unit purchase and renovation costs, rental vouchers and on-going support services from three Connecticut state agencies. The units are owned and managed by the non-profit housing developer and the skilled nursing facility provides the housing case management services. Driven by their founding mission to provide care for persons with HIV/AIDS, Leeway and other skilled nursing organizations have committed themselves to identify gaps in the care continuum and build community partnerships with other AIDS service organizations to enhance the comprehensiveness of medical, behavioral health and social services to this population.

3. Conclusion

The challenge for chronic care for patients with HIV/AIDS in the era of HAART will be to continue to provide appropriate and responsive care and services across the entire, evolving continuum of disease. Whether this widens comprehensive ambulatory case management, home-based care, institutional or post-institutional care, the structure and coordination of care will need to continue to meet the changing needs of a heterogeneous and sometimes vulnerable population. All of these challenges will continue to be compounded by the fact that AIDS remains a highly stigmatizing illness, affecting young individuals and families, with a growing number of medical, behavioral, and psychological co-morbidities which complicate management and create the need for new program and service development. On both a clinical and a policy level, these challenges call for collaboration, flexibility, and cross-disciplinary and cross-agency partnerships in order to respond affectively to this complex, multi-faceted disease as the epidemic widens.

Reference

Abramowitz, S., Obten, N., and Cohen, H. (1998). Measuring case management for families with HIV. *Social Work in Health Care* 27:29-41.

AIDS Housing of Washington. HIV/AIDS Housing Solutions. February, 2003 (http://www.aidshousing.org).

Anderson, M., Paliwoda, J., Kaczynski, R., Schoener, E., Harris, C., Madeja, C., Reid, H., Weber, C., and Trent, C. (2003). Integrating medical and substance abuse treatment for addicts living with HIV/AIDS: Evidence-based nursing practice model. *American Journal of Drug and Alcohol Abuse* 29:847-859.

Bangsburg, D., Tulsky, J., Hecht, F., and Moss, A. (1997). Protease inhibitors in the homeless. *Journal of the American Medical Association* 278:63-65.

Centers for Disease Control. (1991). Mortality attributable to HIV infection/AIDS-United States, 1981-1990. *MMWR* 40:41-44.

Center for Disease Control. (1997). Update: Trends in AIDS incidence, deaths, and prevalence-United States, 1996. *MMWR* 46:165-173.

Center for Disease Control and Prevention. (2000). HIV/AIDS Surveillance Report 12:1-44.

Center for Disease Control. (2001). HIV and AIDS–United States, 1981-2000. *MMWR* 50:430-434.

Cherin, D. A., Huba, G. J., Brief, D. E., and Melchior, L. A. (1998). Evaluation of the Transprofessional Model of Home Health care for HIV/AIDS. *Home Health Care Services Quarterly* 17:55-72.

Cherin, D. A., Simmons, W. J., and Hillary, K. (1998). The Transprofessional Model: Blending intents of terminal care of AIDS. *Home Health Care Services Quarterly* 17:31-54.

Chiasson, M. A., Berenson, L., Li, W., Schwartz, S., Singh, T., Forlenza, S., et al. (1999). Declining HIV/AIDS mortality in New York City. *Journal of Acquired Immune Deficiency Syndrome* 21:59-64.

Chorost, S. (2003). Presentation Titled: Long Term Care; Where Do We Go From Here? New York State AIDS Institute.

Cooper, L. A. and Roter, D. L. (2003). Patient-provider communication: the effect of race and ethnicity on process and outcomes of healthcare. In B. D. Smedley, A.Y. Stith, and A. R. Nelson (Eds.) *Unequal treatment: Confronting racial and ethnic disparities in health care* (pp. 552-593). Washington, D.C.: National Academy Press.

Corless, I. B. and Nicholas, P. K. (2000). Long-term continuum of care for people living with HIV/AIDS. *Journal of Urban Health Bulletin of the New York Academy of Medicine* 77(2):176-186.

De Mello, S. (2000). Connecticut AIDS Residence Coalition. "AIDS Housing is Health Care: A Primer." http://www.ctaidshousing.org/PDFfiles/Primer5.pdf.

Egger, M., Hirschel, B., Francioli, P., Sudre, P., Wirz, M., Flepp, M., et al. (1997). Impact of new antiretroviral combination therapies on HIV infected patients in Switzerland: prospective multicentre study. *BMJ* 315:1194-1199.

Fleishman, J. A. and Crystal, S. (1998). Functional status transitions and survival in HIV disease: Evidence from the AIDS costs and service utilization survey. *Medical Care* 36:533-543.

Foley, F. J., Flannery, J., Graydon, D., Flintoft, G., and Cook, D. (1995). AIDS palliative care: Challenging the palliative paradigm. *Journal of Palliative Care* 11:19-22.

Gomez, M. A. (2004). Enhancing the continuum of care for people living with HIV/AIDS and multiple co-morbididites with home and community-based services in Connecticut. *Yale University Masters Thesis.*

Goulet, J. L., Molde, S., Constantino, J., Gaughan, D., and Selwyn, P. A. (2000). Psychiatric comorbidity and the long-term care of people with AIDS. *Journal of Urban Health: Bulletin of the New York Academy of Medicine* 77(2):213-221.

Greenberg, B., McCorkle, R., Vlahov, D., and Selwyn, P. A. (2000). Palliative care for HIV disease in the era. *Journal of Urban Health Bulletin of the New York Academy of Medicine* 77:150-165.

Grube, B. and Chernesky, R. H. (2001). HIV/AIDS case management tasks and activities: The results of a functional analysis study. *Social Work in Health Care* 32:41-63.

Housing, Health & Wellness Study: A Collaborative Project by Columbia University School of Public Health and Bailey House, October, 2000.

Kravcik, S., Hawley-Foss, N., Victor, G., Angel, J. B., et al. (1997). Causes of death in HIV-infected persons in Ottowa, Ontario, 1984-1995. *Archives of Internal Medicine* 157:2069-2073.

Lee, L., Karon, J., Selik, R., Neal, J., and Fleming, P. (2001). Survival after AIDS diagnosis in adolescents and adults during the treatment era, United States, 1984-1997. *JAMA* 285:1308-1315.

Lehrman, S. E., Gentry, D., Yurchak, B., and Freedman, J. (2001). Outcomes of HIV/AIDS case management in New York. *AIDS Care* 13:481-492.

Lehrman, S., Gimbel, R., Freedman, J., Savicki, K., and Tackley, L. (2002). Development and implementation of an HIV/AIDS case management outcomes assessment programme. *AIDS Care* 14:751-761.

Lynn, L. (1997). An 88-year-old woman facing the end of life. *JAMA* 277:1633-1640.

Mayer, K., Appelbaum, J., Rogers, T., Lo, W., Bradford, J., and Boswell, S. (2001). The evolution of the Fenway Community Health Model. *American Journal of Public Health* 91:892-894.

Merithew, M. A. and Davis-Satterla, L. (2000). Protease inhibitors: Changing the way AIDS case management does business. *Qualitative Health Research* 10:632-645.

Mitchell, J. M. and Anderson, K. H. (2000). Effects of case management and new drugs on Medicaid AIDS spending. *Health Affairs* 19:233-244.

Moore, R., Stanton, D., Gopalan, R., and Chaisson, R. (1994). Racial differences in the use of drug therapy for HIV disease in an urban community. *New England Journal of Medicine* 330:763-768.

Mouton, C., Teno, J. M., Mor, V., and Piette, J. (1997). Communications of preferences for care among human immunodeficiency virus-infected patients. Barriers to informed decisions? *Archives of Family Medicine* 6:342-347.

Oderna, K., Ring, J. and Zalud, S. Yale School of Epidemiology and Public Health. Research paper, 2005.

Oppenhein, S., Hay, J. B., Frederich, M. E., and von Gunten, C. F. (2002). Palliative care in Human Immunodeficiency Virus/Acquired Immunodeficiency Syndrome. In A. M. Berger, R. K. Portenoy, and D.E. Weissman (Eds.). *Palliative Care Supportive Oncology* (2nd ed., pp. 1071-1085). Philadelphia: Lippincott Williams & Wilkins.

Palella, F. J. Jr, Delaney, K. M., Moorman, A. C., et al. (1998). Declining morbidity and mortality among patients with advanced human immunodeficiency virus infection. *New England Journal of Medicine* 338:853-860.

Puoti, M., Spinetti, A., Ghezzi, A., et al. (2001). Mortality from liver disease in patients with HIV infection: a cohort study. *Journal of Acquired Immune Deficiency Syndrome* 24:211-217.

Reester, H., Missmar, R., and Tumlinson, A. Recent Growth in Medicaid Home and Community-Based Service Waivers. The Health Strategies Consultancy for the Kaiser Commission on Medicaid and the Uninsured, April (2004). Pg. 1.

Sansone, R. G. and Frengley, J. D. (2000). Impact of HAART on causes of death of persons with late-stage AIDS. *Journal of Urban Health* 77:165-175.

Selwyn, P. A. (1996). HIV therapy in the real world. *AIDS* 10:1591-1593

Selwyn, P. A. and Arnold, R. (1998) From fate to tragedy: the changing meanings of life, death, and AIDS. *Annals of Internal Medicine* 129:899-902.

Selwyn, P. A., Goulet, J. L., Molde, S., et al. (2000). HIV as a chronic disease: long-term care for patients with HIV at a dedicated skilled nursing facility. *Journal of Urban Health* 77:187-203.

Silha S. Building Compassion; The History of Bailey-Boushay House, from Breaking New Ground: Developing Innovative AIDS Care Residences, Lieberman, Betsy; Donald P. Chamberlain, AIDS Housing Washington, 1993.

Sorensen, J. L., Dilley, J., London, J., Okin, R. L., Delucchi, K. L., and Phibbs, C. (2003). Case management for substance abusers with HIV/AIDS: A randomized clinical trial. *American Journal of Drug and Alcohol Abuse* 29:133-150.

Sowell, R. L. (1995). Community-Based HIV case management: Challenges and opportunities. *Journal of the Association of Nurses in AIDS Care* 6:33-40.

Valdez, H., Chowdhry, T. K., Asaad, R., et al. (2001). Changing spectrum of mortality due to HIV:analysis of 260 deaths during 1995-1999. *Clinical Infectious Diseases* 32:1487-93.

Weinstein, M. C., Toy, E. L., Sanberg, E. A., Neumann, P. J., Evans, J. S., Kuntz, K. M., Graham, J. D. and Hammitt, J. K. (2001). Modeling for health care and other policy decisions: Uses, roles, & validity. *Value in Health* 4:348-361.

Wenger, N. S., Kanouse, D. E., Collins, R. L., et al. (2001). End-of-life discussions and preferences among persons with HIV. *JAMA* 285:2880-2887.

Wong, T., Chiasson, A., Reggy, A., Simonds, R. J., Heffess, K., and Loo, V. (2000). Antiretroviral therapy and declining AIDS mortality in New York City. *Journal of Urban Health* 77:492-500.

www.CDC.gov/hiv

http://www.cms.hhs.gov/medicaid/1915c/default.asp

http://documents.csh.org/documents/ct/loct-CTPG-1-intro.htm#1

7
Palliative Care and Chronic Obstructive Lung Disease

Manoj Karwa MD*, Alpana Chandra MD,
and Adnan Mirza MD

Chronic Obstructive Pulmonary Disease (COPD) is a major public health problem in the United States and throughout the world with a global prevalence estimated at 9.3 per 1000 males and 7.3 per 1000 females (all ages). (Vital and Health Statistics, 1996; Murray and Lopez, 1997). COPD was ranked as the sixth most common cause of death worldwide in 1990, and the Global Burden of Disease Study predicted that it would become the third most common cause by 2020 (Lopez and Murray, 1998). In 2003, an estimated 10.7 million adults in the U.S. were reported as having physician diagnosed COPD. However data from the NHANES III (National Health and Nutrition Evaluation Survey) estimated that approximately 24 million adults in the U.S. have evidence of impaired lung function, indicating an underdiagnosis of COPD especially in its milder forms which are most amenable to treatment. It is estimated that there may be 16 million people in the U.S. currently diagnosed with COPD (Hilleman *et al.*, 2000; NCHS, 2002). Mortality and morbidity is significant in patients who have severe COPD, are elderly and have acute exacerbations of COPD requiring hospitalization or ICU admission. According to estimates by the National Heart Lung and Blood Instiute, in 2004 the total annual expenditure for COPD in the U.S. was $37.2 billion, including $20.9 billion for hospital costs and treatment of the disease and $1,613 billion in indirect costs such as work loss. (National Institutes of Health. National Heart, Lung and Blood Institute, 2002). Despite the relatively high prevalence, morbidity, and mortality, end-of-life care such as hospice placement occurs in only a small percentage of patients with COPD.

MANOJ KARWA • Assistant Professor of Medicine, Division of Critical Care Medicine, Gold Zone first floor, Montefiore Medical Center, 111th East 210th Street, Bronx, New York 10467. ALPANA CHANDRA • ADNAN MIRZA • Fellow in Critical Care Medicine, Division of Critical Care Medicine, Gold Zone first floor, Montefiore Medical Center, 111th East 210th Street, Bronx, New York 10467 and *Corresponding author: Assistant Professor of Medicine, Division of Critical Care Medicine, Gold Zone first floor, Montefiore Medical Center, 111th East 210th Street, Bronx, New York 10467.

1. Definition, Pathophysiology and Classification of COPD

COPD is a slowly progressive disease in which the airways are obstructed and there is accelerated loss of lung function over time. The American Thoracic Society incorporates chronic bronchitis, emphysema and airway hyper-reactivity in its definition. The Global Initiative for Chronic Obstructive Lung Disease (GOLD), a collaborative project of the National Institute of Heart, Lung and Blood Diseases and the World Health Organization, highlights the progressive nature of COPD. GOLD defines COPD as a disease state characterized by airflow limitation that is not fully reversible and associated with an abnormal inflammatory response of the lungs to inhalation of toxic substances (Barnes, 2000; Pauwels *et al.*, 2004; American Thoracic Society and European Respiratory Society, 2004). Over 80% of COPD cases are due to tobacco use or exposure. Patients with COPD are plagued by symptoms of cough, increased sputum production, and exertional dyspnea disproportionate to their age and activity level. With continued exposure patients develop increased exercise intolerance, dyspnea at rest, and an overall decrease in their quality of life.

In COPD, inflammation of lung parenchyma and small airways, causes increased mucous production, airway hyper-reactivity, and emphysematous changes within the lungs. These factors cause irreversible expiratory flow limitation and hyperinflation of the lungs, lessening the efficiency of the diaphragm in inspiration and expiration of the lungs. These features contribute to ineffective ventilation and gas exchange. Over time secondary pulmonary hypertension and cor pulmonale (right sided heart failure) develop (Sullivan *et al.*, 2000).

Hyperinflation, often called air trapping, refers to an increase in the volume of air in the lungs resulting from the inability to fully exhale, or expiratory flow limitation. The sudden and abrupt accumulation of air contributes to the sensation of respiratory discomfort and breathlessness. Dynamic hyperinflation is hyperinflation that is associated with any physical activity— walking, climbing stairs or any other tasks that increase breathing demands. Currently both the ATS and GOLD agree that cough, sputum production, dyspnea, or exposure to risk factors be considered in making the diagnosis of COPD. In addition, there should be evidence of irreversible airflow limitation by the FEV1/FVC ratio ≤ 70% after use of a bronchodilator medication. (FEV1 = forced expiratory volume in one second, FVC = forced vital capacity). The ATS/ERS (European Respiratory Society) severity score leave as to some extent does help predict health status, utilization of health-care resources, development of exacerbation, and mortality. These scoring systems should be used as tools and not substitute for clinical judgment in evaluating the severity of disease (Table 7.1).

TABLE 7.1. Comparison of the ATS/ERS and gold scoring systems (3, 77, 85, 91)

Severity or stage	ATS / ERS	Gold
At risk or stage 0	FEV1/FVC >70 %, FEV1 ≥80% Patients who: Smoke or have exposure to pollutants Have cough, sputum, dypnea Have family history of respiratory disease	Normal spirometery Chronic symptoms of cough, or sputum production
Mild or stage I	FEV1/FVC ≤ 70%, FEV1 ≥ 80%	• FEV1/FVC < 70% • FEV1 ≥ 80% predicted • with or without chronic symptoms (cough, sputum production)
Moderate or stage II	FEV1/FVC ≤ 0.7, FEV1 50–80	• FEV1/FVC < 70% • 50% ≤ FEV1 < 80% predicted • with or without chronic symptoms (cough, sputum production)
Severe or stage III	FEV1/FVC ≤0.7, FEV1 30–50	• FEV1/FVC < 70% • 30% ≤ FEV1 < 50% predicted • with or without chronic symptoms (cough, sputum production)
Very severe or stage IV	FEV1/FVC ≤ 0.7, FEV1 < 30	• FEV1/FVC < 70% • FEV1 < 30% predicted or FEV1 < 50% predicted plus chronic respiratory failure

2. Natural History of the Disease

2.1. Decline in Lung Function

In adults over 30 years, FEV1 normally declines by about 30 ml per year, but this doubles in patients with COPD and active heavy smokers (Anthonisen *et al.*, 2002; Anthonisen *et al.*, 2005; Guidelines Group of the Standards of Care Committee of the BTS, 1997; James and Hallenbeck, 2003). The onset of symptoms such as, exertional dyspnea is variable, but often does not occur until the FEV_1 has decreased to a range of 40% to 59% of the predicted normal value (American Thoracic Society and European Respiratory Society, 2004; Guidelines Group of the Standards of Care Committee of the BTS, 1997; Pauwels *et al.*, 2004; Sutherland and Cherniack, 2004). This may explain the underdiagnosis in the earliest stages of COPD. The stage of the disease portends the prognosis, and follow-up data from two longitudinal studies indicate that moderate and severe stages of the disease are associated with higher mortality rate and risk of death. (Anthonisen, 1986; Mannino et al., 2003). (Figure 7.1 and 7.2) When the FEV1 goes below 1L, the mortality rate is in the range of 50% at five years. (Fletcher and Peto, 1977).

2.2. Acute Exacerbations of Disease

The progressive decline in lung function in COPD is often interrupted by a debilitating increase in symptoms, requiring hospitalization, commonly known as an acute exacerbation of COPD (AECOPD). AECOPD generally occurs at GOLD stage II disease or higher, is usually caused by viral or bacterial infections, and heralded by an increase in symptoms (Fagon and Chastre, 1996). A decline in FEV1 may or may not correlate with the frequency of exacerbations (Decramer et al., 1997; Kessler et al., 1999; Osman et al., 1997). However, studies do suggest that early mortality is correlated with AECOPD requiring hospitalization.

Patients with acute exacerbations admitted to an ICU face a hospital mortality rate as high as 24%. For patients 65 or older, the mortality rate is 30% at the time of hospital discharge, increasing to 59% at one year. There were findings in a prospective study by Seneff and associates of ICU admissions

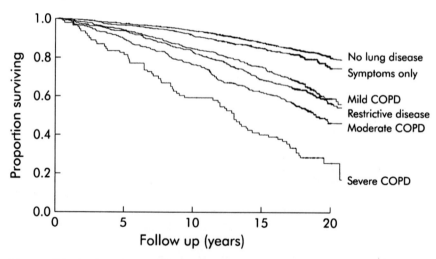

FIGURE 7.1. Kaplan-Meier curve for death among 5542 participants stratified by degree of lung function impairment From the National Health and Nutrition Examination Survey 1971–5 and follow up to 1992. With permission from Mannino, D.M., et al., Lung function and mortality in the United States: data from the First National Health and Nutrition Examination Survey follow up study. Thorax, 2003. 58(5): p. 388-93. (68)

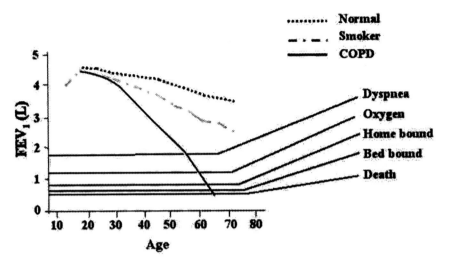

FIGURE 7.2. Natural History of COPD compared to smokers without COPD, and 'normals'. Dyspnea, need for oxygen, sedentary life style and mortality are correlated with the FEV1. Adapted with permission from Fletcher, C. and R. Peto, The natural history of chronic airflow obstruction. Br Med J, 1977. 1(6077): p. 1645-8. (34)

for acute exacerbation of COPD. Of interest, development of non-respiratory organ system dysfunction was shown to be the major predictor of hospital mortality and 180-day outcomes. (Seneff *et al.*, 1995)

Almagro, in a prospective study of 135 consecutive patients admitted for AECOPD, showed that mortality at six months, one year and two years was 13.4%, 22%, and 35.6% respectively. Moreover, hospitalization for AECOPD was an independent predictor of mortality for subsequent hospitalizations. The risk increased with the number of previous hospitalizations. (Almagro, 2002) In a retrospective study of a cohort of 166 patients, admitted for AECOPD and requiring mechanical ventilation, 28% died in the hospital. The need for invasive mechanical ventilation for more than 72 hours was an independent predictor of poor outcome. The study was conducted by Nevins and Epstein at New England Medical Center, Tufts University School of Medicine. (Nevins and Epstein, 2001)

2.3. Quality of Life

According to the National Health Information Survey (NHIS) 1980-1996, between 1994 and 1996, 57.5% of patients with self reported COPD (no spirometric testing was employed), 38.6% had activity limitation, and 8% reported COPD associated activity limitation (Mannino *et al.*, 2002). In the NHANES III, between 1991-1994, of the patients with spirometric evidence of moderate COPD (FEV1/FVC ≤ 70%, and FEV1 < 80%), 18% had difficulty walking a quarter of a mile, 13.9% had difficulty lifting or carrying 10 pounds, and 7% needed help in handling routine chores.

As only supplemental oxygen therapy improves survival, and smoking cessation is the only intervention that retards decline in lung function in COPD, it is obvious that most other treatments are aimed at improving quality of life. Although physiologic variables, to a great extent, correlate with severity of disease and mortality, many patients with only minimal disease have a disproportionate number of symptoms and functional limitation. This is partly due to the multifaceted nature of COPD, with patients not only having airflow limitation but under nutrition, other existing co-morbid illnesses, dynamic hyperinflation, and pulmonary hypertension. Thus patient's perceptions and ability to adapt, largely define the quality of life. Ultimately patients are more concerned with symptom relief and improvement in their functional status.

Commonly used respiratory disease specific quality-of-life questionnaires include the Chronic Respiratory Disease Questionnaire (CRQ), Pulmonary Functional Status and Dyspnea Questionnaire (PFSDQ), Pulmonary Function Status Scale (PFSS), St. George's Respiratory Questionnaire (SGRQ), and the Seattle Obstructive Lung Disease Questionnaire (SOLQ). The description of these instruments is beyond the scope of this chapter and the reader is referred to several excellent reviews (Guyatt et al., 1993; Mahler et al., 1992; Testa and Simonson, 1996).

Several studies have shown that patients with COPD have both poorer general and disease-specific Health Related Quality of Life (HRQOL) scores (Ferrer et al., 1997; Hajiro et al., 1998; Mahler et al., 1992; Mahler and Mackowiak, 1995). Breathlessness and pain were described as "very distressing" in the last year of life in 76% and 56% of patients with COPD respectively, cough in 46% and anorexia in 15% (Edmonds et al., 2001). Poorer HRQOL scores have been correlated with increased number of hospitalizations and mortality (Fan et al., 2002). Anxiety, nutritional status, and marital status have all been implicated as predictors of mortality, and more so as disease severity increases (Santo Tomas and Varkey, 2004). Domingo-Salvany et al. followed a cohort of 321 male COPD patients over five years and found that the SGRQ, as well as the SF-36 health survey score, independently correlated with both all-cause and respiratory mortality. Patients with ATS stage III COPD had a 60% survival, stage II a 73% survival, and stage I an 89% survival at four years (Salvany, 2002). (Figure 7.3) The investigators also demonstrated that a four point increase in the SGRQ score was associated with an increase in risk of global mortality of 5.1%.

2.4. Causes of Death

Major causes of death in COPD include acute or chronic respiratory failure, pulmonary infection, heart failure, pulmonary embolism, cardiac arrhythmia, and lung cancer. A prospective cohort study of 135 patients admitted for AECOPD found that the causes of death were respiratory failure (50%),

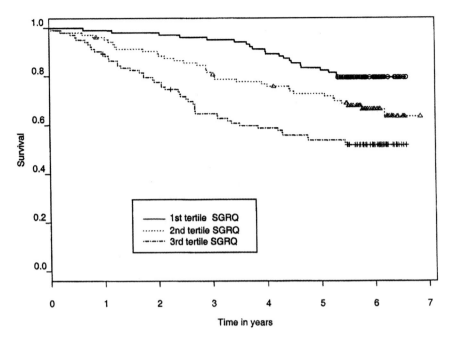

FIGURE 7.3. SGRQ tertiles and survival probabilities in COPD patients. Reprinted with permission from Salvany AD *et al.*, Health-related Quality of Life and Mortality in Male Patients with Chronic Obstructive Pulmonary Disease. Am J Respir Crit Care Med 2002: 166; 680–685. (82)

cardiovascular disease (19%), cancer (6%), and unknown / other (25%). Chronic heart failure was the most frequent associated comorbidity (OR 2.3). (Hansell *et al.*, 2003; Meyer *et al.*, 2002; Zielinski *et al.*, 1997).

In 2003, 122,283 patients died of COPD and 52% of deaths were in women. This was the fourth consecutive year in which the number of COPD deaths in women exceeded those in men. Although COPD causes almost as many deaths as lung cancer, knowledge of the impact of COPD in the late stages of illness is limited. In one study Elkington and associates assessed the healthcare needs of COPD patients in the last year of life by means of a retrospective survey of the informants of 399 COPD deaths in four London health programs (Elkington *et al.*, 2005). Symptoms, day-to-day functioning, contact with health and social services were assessed. Based on the reports, 98% of patients were breathless all the time or some of the time in the last year of life; other symptoms present all the time or sometimes included fatigue or weakness (96%), low mood (77%), and pain (70%). Patients lacked surveillance and received insufficient services from primary and secondary providers in the year before they died. The investigators also noted the absence of palliative care programs and the need to address issues such as uncontrolled symptoms and end-of-life planning (Elkington *et al.*, 2005).

2.5. *Patterns of Functional Decline and Death*

The pattern of declining function is not correlated well with FEV1, although the probability of death is. Early reports on the natural history of COPD as it relates to FEV1 showed a strong correlation. (Fletcher and Peto, 1977) (Figure 7.2) This is, however, an oversimplification and represents an average of all the patients studied. Not all patients follow the classical trajectory outlined. In fact decline in FEV1 is more likely to be quite varied from patient to patient. (Figure 7.4) The pattern of death is best described as the entry-

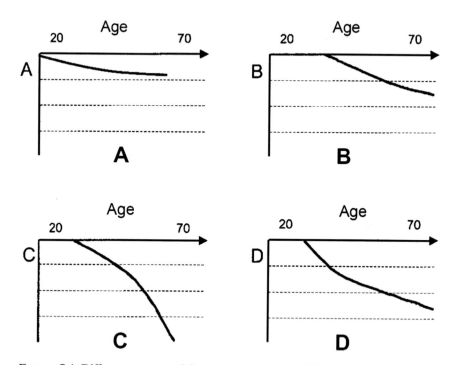

FIGURE 7.4. Different patterns of functional decline in COPD: shows four examples of the various courses that individual COPD patients may follow. Panel A illustrates an individual who has cough and sputum production, but never develops abnormal lung function (as defined in this Report). Panel B illustrates an individual who develops abnormal lung function but who may never come to diagnosis. Panel C illustrates a person who develops abnormal lung function around age 50, then progressively deteriorates over about 15 years and dies of respiratory failure at age 65. Panel D illustrates an individual who develops abnormal lung function in mid-adult life and continues to deteriorate gradually but never develops respiratory failure and does not die as a result of COPD. With permission from Pauwels RA, Buist AS, Calverley PM, *et al*, the GOLD Scientific Committee. Global strategy for the diagnosis, management, and prevention of chronic obstructive pulmonary disease, 2004 Update. NHLBI/WHO Global Initiative for Chronic Obstructive Lung Disease (GOLD) Workshop summary. Available at www.goldcopd.com accessed December 2004. (77)

reentry pattern. Here patients have sudden acute declines followed by substantial improvements, while still having an overall downward trend in function,in contrast to the trajectories for cancer and frailty. (Lukert, 1994) (Figure 7.5).

Lunney *et al.* analyzed the functional decline of 4190 decedents who died within 12 months of an initial interview for the period between 1981-1987 (Lunney *et al.*, 2003). Decedents with organ failure (COPD and heart failure) were compared to decedents with cancer, frailty, and victims of sudden death. Decedents of the organ failure group had a more erratic decline when compared to the cancer group, and sudden death group. (Figure 7.5) Cancer decedents had a much steeper decline in level of function during the last three months of life when compared to the other three groups. The organ failure group had more functional limitation in the first half of the year than those in the cancer group. Organ failure decedents were more likely to be elderly compared to the cancer and sudden death group, and the elderly in all groups were four times more likely to require assistance

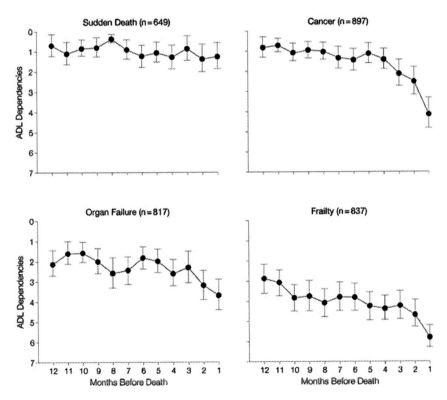

FIGURE 7.5. Various patterns of functional decline towards death. Reprinted with permission from Lunney JR *et al.*, Patterns of functional decline at the end of life, JAMA, 2003; 289(18), 2387-2392. (58)

(Lunney *et al.*, 2003). These observations are significant in that the pattern of functional decline is less predictable in patients with COPD. This in turn influences one's expectancy of death, need for hospice care, and advance directive planning.

These observations have been reinforced in a study done by Teno *et al.* (Teno *et al.*, 2001). Using a mortality followback survey of the decedents next of kin and death certificates from the National Centers for health statistics 1993, they analyzed the pattern of functional decline (days of difficulty with activities of daily living, and mobility), as well as the the use of hospice services, and site of death in 3,614 decedents during the last year of life. They compared decedents of cancer, heart failure, COPD, cerebral vascular accidents, and diabetes mellitus. Decedents of cancer were more likely to have received hospice services and to die at home than the other groups. Decedents of COPD were the most likely to die in a hospital. Cancer decedents had a higher level of function than those in other groups at one year prior to death, but at five months prior to death the cancer group experienced a much steeper decline in function. (Figure 7.6) More precipitous functional decline correlated with hospice involvement and dying at home (Figure 7.7).

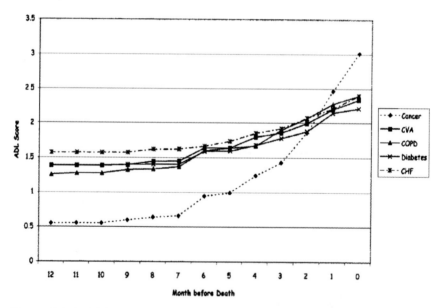

FIGURE 7.6. Activities of Daily living scores one year prior to dying in cancer and non cancer patients. Reprinted with permission Teno JM *et al.*, Dying Trajectory in the Last Year of Life: Does Cancer Trajectory Fit Other Diseases? Journal of Palliative Medicine; 2001, 4(4):457-464. (96)

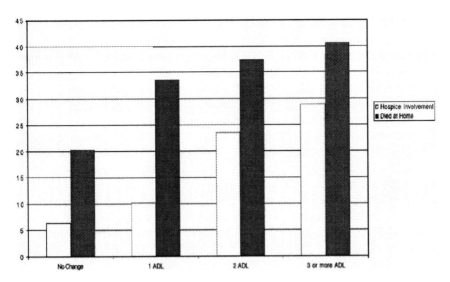

FIGURE 7.7. Correlation between Activities of daily living, hospice involvement and site of death Reprinted with permission from Teno JM *et al.*, Dying Trajectory in the Last Year of Life: Does Cancer Trajectory Fit Other Diseases? Journal Of Palliative Medicine; 2001, 4(4):457-464. (96)

3. Burden of COPD

Disability and death from COPD is increasing. (Costello *et al.*, 1997; James *et al.*, 2005; Manning, 2000; Yach *et al.*, 2004) COPD has already risen to become the fourth most common cause of death and is the only common cause of death in the U.S. whose prevalence has increased over the past 20 years. (Hurd, 2000; Mannino *et al.*, 2000)

In 2000 there were a total of 7,997,000 outpatient visits, 1,549,000 emergency room visits, and a total of 726,000 hospitalizations for patients with COPD. (Mannino *et al.*, 2000) According to the National Health Interview Survey, of patients having COPD, 64.6% were employed, 18.4% reported any limitation of activity, and 7 to 8% had COPD related limitation of activity and difficulty handling routine needs of daily living (Vital and health statistics, 1996). COPD is responsible for work loss of approximately $9.9 billion per year in the U.S.

COPD is a major cause of chronic disability and predicted to become the fifth most common cause of disability in the world by 2020. COPD is a major cause of health care expenditure that now exceeds the costs associated with asthma by more than a factor of three (Sin *et al.*, 2002; Strassels *et al.*, 2001; Sullivan *et al.*, 2000). In a survey of 3,265 patients and 905 physicians, Halpern *et al.*, calculated that the indirect cost of COPD was $,1527 (from work loss) and the total cost was $5,646. When analyzing direct costs, the annual cost of health care utilization per patient was $4,120, and the highest cost of any individual resource being that of inpatient hospitalizations ($2891). (Halpern *et al.*, 2003) An interpretation of the study is that COPD is more costly to the health care system and society than to patients with COPD alone.

Total treatment cost is highly correlated with disease severity. A pharmacoeconomic analysis was conducted by Hilleman and associates at the Creighton University School of Pharmacy, Omaha. Healthcare resource utilization and costs were identified through chart review and stratified using the ATS criteria. They calculated that patients treated for stage III COPD had the highest average cost ($10,812 per patient per year), and patients with stage I COPD had the lowest cost ($1,683 per patient per year) (Hilleman *et al.*, 2000). Stage III patients had an average of 3.2 hospitalizations per year compared to 0.3 of patients with stage I disease. Furthermore over five years the mortality for patients with stage III disease was 33% compared to 0% and 17% of patients with Stage I and II disease respectively. (Table 7.2) Of the $ 20.9 billion spent in direct medical costs for COPD only 3.3% was spent on home health care services and 13.4 % on nursing home care. (National Institutes of Health. National Heart, Lung and Blood Institute, 2004)

4. Palliative Care

4.1. Insights from the SUPPORT Trial and Prognostication

As we have seen there is an increase in mortality with the severity of the COPD as measured by spirometry, age, smoking status, body mass index, number of AECOPD, need for mechanical ventilation, HRQOL measurement

TABLE 7.2. Breakdown of costs of care for COPD patients by severity of disease

Cost categories	Severity of COPD		
	Stage I†	Stage II†	Stage III†
Initial drug acquisition cost	$ 299 (18)	$ 529 (11)	$ 634 (6)
Add-on drug acquisition cost	$ 213 (13)	$ 191 (4)	$ 132 (1)
Total drug acquisition cost	$ 512 (31)	$ 720 (14)	$ 766 (7)
Oxygen therapy	0 (0)	$ 699 (14)	$ 2,012 (19)
Laboratory/diagnostic test cost	$ 345 (20)	$ 493 (10)	$ 610 (6)
Clinic visit cost	$ 82 (5)	$ 148 (3)	$ 171 (2)
Emergency department visit cost	$ 62 (4)	$ 319 (6)	$ 483 (4)
Hospitalization cost	$ 680 (40)	$2,658 (53)	$ 6,770 (63)
Total cost	$1,681 (100)	$5,037 (100)	$ 10,812 (100)

Costs are presented as per patient per year (percentage of total cost). †p, 0.01 for each cost variable and total cost across the three severities of COPD. Reprinted with permission from Hilleman DE *et al.*, Pharmacoeconomic evaluation of COPD. Chest 2000; I 18:1278-1285. (46)

TABLE 7.3. Prognostic factors in chronic obstructive pulmonary disease

FEV1	54% 5-year survival. Mean FEV1 1.04 ± 0.41. **(27, 68, 77)**
Age	Mortality higher in the elderly. Mean age 61 ± 8 yrs. Mean FEV1 36.1 ± 11.4%. **(5, 68, 71)**
PaO2	Increased mortality when PaO2 < 55 untreated. **(74)**
BMI	24% 5-year survival for BMI < 20 kg/m2. Mean FEV1 31% ± 12. All required LTOT. **(17)**
Dyspnea	SGRQ and SOLDQ correlated with mortality independent of FEV1 **(82)**
Apache II	Apache II score on admission to general medicine ward correlated with death at 3 years. 50% mortality at 3 years for Apache II > 20 **(27, 79)**
Hospital admission to ICU for AECOPD with respiratory failure	Unselected COPD patients administrative database. In-hospital mortality 2.5% **(76)** 22% mortality at 1 year after hospitalization **(2)**
Hospital admission to ICU for AECOPD with respiratory failure	15% in-hospital ICU mortality rate. 46% required invasive mechanical ventilation. Nonsurvivors mean Apache II 25.6 ± 8.7. **(73)**
BODE index	Better predictor of mortality than FEV1 **(16)**

scores, and other physiological variables. (Table 7.3) Despite this seemingly abundant and convincing data, identifying patients with COPD who are at risk of dying with in six months is far from precise.

The landmark investigation, Study to Understand Prognoses and Preferences for Outcomes and Risks of Treatment (SUPPORT), offers great insight into the outcomes of hospitalized COPD patients, in terms of six month survival, patient preferences about advance directives, practices surrounding advance directives, patient physician communication, and use of hospital resources prior to death. For example, Connors and associates studied a prospective cohort of 1,016 adult patients enrolled in SUPPORT; all were hospitalized with an acute exacerbation of COPD. The likelihood of a poor outcome was markedly increased after acute exacerbation particularly in association with a $PaCO_2$ of 50mmHg or more, indicating an excess of carbon dioxide in the blood which can lead to hypercarbic respiratory failure (Connors et al., 1996; Knaus et al., 1995).

In a separate analysis of SUPPORT phase I and II, of patients with COPD who died within one year of enrollment, Lynn et al., found that 15% to 25% of the patients spent the last six months of life in the hospital. It was only in the last few days that the model was able to predict a lower survival; despite this there was still a 30% likelihood of surviving past six months (Connors et al., 1996; Lynn et al., 2000).

In a study using data from SUPPORT phase I and II, Fox et al., tested the utility of applying five general and two disease-specific clinical criteria (based on the then National Hospice Organizations criteria for hospice eligibility) for identifying a survival prognosis of six months or less after surviving hospitalization for a serious illness. The five general criteria used were readmission to a hospital within two months, home care after discharge, dependency in three activities of daily living, weight loss of more than five pounds within two months, and an albumin level of less than 25 g/L. The two COPD-specific clinical criteria used were presence of cor pulmonale and a reduced blood oxygen level (PaO2 of 55 mm Hg or less) while receiving oxygen therapy. Three sets of combined criteria (broad, intermediate and narrow inclusion) were used, aimed at providing low, medium, or high thresholds for hospice eligibility. Broad inclusion required only one of the seven clinical criteria, intermediate required three, and narrow required five. Of a total of 900 patients with COPD, 74% survived for longer than six months. Of the 900 patients approximately 30%, expressed a preference for palliative care. When survival was analyzed using the combination criteria 68% of patients in the broad inclusion set survived more than six months, 67% in the intermediate set, and 50% in the narrow set. Only 3.3% were actually discharged to hospice and the large majority of these patients died within six months. Thus the greatest prognostic factor for survival less than six months was discharge to hospice (which was not part of the criteria tested). The authors concluded that using criteria to predict six month mortality and hospice eligibility were not so much inaccurate as they were unrealistic for this patient population (Connors et al., 1996; Fox et al., 1999).

The last year of life for patients with COPD is markedly different in comparison to patients who die of cancer. As described by Teno et al. and Lunney et al., COPD patients experience a pattern of dying marked by periods when they are seriously ill and recover. (Figures 7.5-7.7). Although the overall prognosis of these patients is considered poor, even in comparison to some terminal cancer patients, they tend to live for variable periods of time in a state of ill health. Their death is less predictable, and often may come suddenly and unpredictably. This has important implications in regards to prognostication for hospice services. It also has psycho-social effects on the patient in that they may not have time to realize and accept death as natural part of their life cycle. In addition families of the patient may not have sufficient time to bereave and acclimate to their loss.

4.2. Advance Directives in COPD

Since predicting survival of less than one year or six months is inaccurate, discussion about advance directives can be challenging for the physician. Patient autonomy about such decisions is both in line with the principles of palliative care as well as with the patient's preferences. In one study by Heffner et al., 88.6% of patients in a pulmonary rehabilitation program wanted to know about advance directives (AD), yet only 19% had discussions with their physicians and only 14.3% thought that their physicians knew their wishes (Heffner et al., 1996). In the SUPPORT trial only 38% of COPD patients showed preference for do not resuscitate (DNR) orders, but 78% expressed wishes for comfort care measures, saying that they 'would rather die' than be attached to a ventilator 'all the time' (Lynn *et al.*, 2000). Approximately 46% of all DNR orders for the patients in SUPPORT (including patients with COPD) were made within two days of death. This highlights the lack of any gradual transition from active care to palliative hospice care and reflects the erratic dying trajectory of these patients. The failure of the SUPPORT interventions to improve physician patient communications, timing of DNR orders, physician knowledge of patients wishes, and to decrease the days spent in the ICU on ventilators is not surprising in the case of COPD for this very reason. Thus one may adopt the philosophy that palliative care should not necessarily preclude life-sustaining therapy in the case of COPD. However, in keeping with this line of care one should note that approximately 25% to 30% of patients have significant pain, 70% to 85% have dyspnea, and about 20% have confusion, all of which increased closer to time of death (Edmonds *et al.*, 2001; Lynn et al., 2000).

Discussions about AD should address patient preferences for cardio-pulmonary resuscitation (CPR) and mechanical ventilation, discussions with family members if allowable, provisions for surrogate decision making, alternatives to aggressive therapies, education about the nature of COPD and inaccuracies about prognostication, and assurance of adequate symptom control. The caregiver should keep in mind the patient's perception of discussions about AD. Physicians tend to mark the discussion as an operational tool directing which therapies are to be used and which not, and fear the removal of hope. However the patient may regard this as an event signaling their preparation for death and fortifying their psychosocial, emotional, and spiritual needs.

4.3. Delivery of Palliative Care in COPD

Palliative care for end-stage COPD includes assessment and management of the patient's suffering and concerns on several different fronts. These include alleviating physical suffering, providing both emotional and spiritual support, as well as keeping a constant line of communication for both the patients and their families. Thus the emphasis shifts from focusing on abnormal laboratory values and more on the quality of life. The delivery of this multifaceted type of care through the use of comprehensive teams employing physicians, social workers, chaplains, and psychologists, has met with some success in improving the patient's dyspnea, anxiety, spiritual well being and sleep quality. (Rabow *et al.*, 2004)

Probably the most disabling symptom for the patient with end stage COPD is the sensation of dyspnea which is often not explicable only on the basis of physiological factors (American Thoracic society, 1999; Sorenson, 2000). Dyspnea assessment is subjective but can be graded according to the Borg 12 point scale ranging from 0 for 'nothing at all' to 12 'maximal dyspnea'

(Borg, 1990; Sorenson, 2000). Sixty percent of the SUPPORT patients had severe dyspnea in the last two months of life and 90% during the last three days (Lynn et al., 2000). The main stay of therapy for dyspnea has been the use of opioids. Opioids help in decreasing all phases of ventilation, which correlates directly with the level of dyspnea, as well as directly decreasing the sensation. They have also shown to be of benefit in reducing exertional dyspnea (Light et al., 1989). In a meta-analysis of randomized double blind placebo controlled trials of opioids for dyspnea, Jennings et al. found a positive and greater effect of relief of dyspnea with the use of both oral and parenetral opioids compared to nebulized opioids. Additionally there was no difference noted between the use of single versus multiple dosing regimens (Jennings et al., 2002). But there is the danger of decreasing ventilation to life threatening levels.

Coinciding with the sensation of dyspnea is the feeling of anxiety and depression (Light et al., 1989). The SUPPORT trial as well as other studies examining HRQOL in patients with COPD attest to this. In SUPPORT patients had low levels of both anxiety and depression, which became more prevalent in the population closer to death. Low-dose benzodiazipines help in the management of anxiety but have no direct effect on the sensation of dyspnea. At least one study has shown that use of sedation for palliation of symptoms is not necessarily associated with a lessening of prognosis (Cherny and Portenoy, 1994). Both anxiolytics and antidepressants do have a thera-peutic rationale in dyspnea treatment but convincing evidence for the efficacy is scant (Argyropoulou et al., 1993; Mannino et al., 2000; Mitchell-Heggs et al., 1980; Smoller et al., 1998). Oxygen is another therapy widely used in the palliation of dyspnea, however many of the trials have focused on improvement of physiological variables as opposed to alleviation of breath-lessness. Existing trials show a varied outcome in the reduction of breath-lessness however (Booth et al., 2004). Furthermore oxygen therapy is one of the few therapies that has been shown to improve survival in patients with COPD who have oxygen deficiency (hypoxia). (Nocturnal Oxygen Therapy Trial Group, 1980)

The use of forced air via a simple fan has proven to be of some benefit in alleviating dyspnea (Mannino, 2002; Spence et al., 1993). Chest wall vibra-tion, delivered in phase with the respiratory cycle, vagotomy, acupuncture and acupressure have been tried but there are too few published studies to support their routine use (Benditt, 2000; Berglund et al., 1971; Jobst et al., 1986; Maa et al., 1997; Sibuya et al., 1994). There is an increasing trend in the enrollment of patients with severe COPD into pulmonary rehabilitation programs although they have not shown to decrease mortality or baseline physiology, rehabilitation does increase exercise tolerance, help alleviating baseline and exertional dyspnea, and improve HRQOL scores. In addition the programs serve as a unique setting for the initiation of discussion of advanced directives. (Heffner, 2000)

Noninvasive ventilation has usually been used as a curative intervention for certain varieties of respiratory failure but might also be useful as a palliative measure for the relief of dyspnea. (Cazzolli and Oppenheimer, 1996) While most medications used to treat dyspnea have the potential to reduce the life span by reducing the respiratory drive and causing hypercarbic respiratory failure, noninvasive ventilation may produce just the opposite effect by supporting respiration and prolonging life as well as relieving symptoms of dyspnea. This might also be used to support patients with advanced COPD during acute exacerbations who reject mechanical ventilation. However a prerequisite for its use is that the patient be alert enough to comprehend its use and be able to cooperate as well as tolerate the therapy. With non invasive positive pressure ventilation (NPPV) verbal communication can be maintained, whereas this is severely impaired with endotracheal intubation and can generate fear, anxiety and feelings of isolation in the dying (Hansen-Flaschen, 2000). NPPV has been shown to improve the quality of life, impact on neuropsychological function, and improve sleep quality (Elliott et al., 1992; Perrin et al., 1997; Strumpf et al., 1991). Hence NPPV is a novel option for palliation easily rendered by a well-trained and competent respiratory staff. The use of NPPV is an emerging palliative therapy for patients with severe COPD although convincing evidence for its routine use is not present.

Excess secretions, while not the most common pulmonary symptom in dying patients, are nevertheless troublesome. If significant in volume they can cause airway obstruction, trigger a persistent cough, increase dyspnea and interfere with sleep. Atropine sulfate, hyoscyamine sulfate (Levsin), and hyoscine hydrobromide (scopolamine) have all been used to some degree of effectiveness and atropine drops administered to the back of the throat in terminally ill patients provide fairly rapid relief from excess secretions. Broad-spectrum antibiotics, bronchodilators and mucolytics have been the primary therapeutic intervention for exacerbation of COPD and might also be useful otherwise. Airway clearance devices are used to clear the airways of mucus for the purpose of improving breathing and reducing the chances for respiratory infections to develop. For example, exhaling through a positive expiratory (PEP) device creates oscillation in airway pressures. The flutter helps to mobilize secretions. PEP devices promote mucus clearance in part by preventing airway closure and increasing collateral ventilation. Relatively new, intra-pulmonary percussive ventilation (IPV) has been found to be as effective as chest physiotherapy and aerosol therapy in enhancing sputum production. Approximately 20% of the patients in the SUPPORT trial had severe pain with the incidence increasing as death approached (Classens, 2000). Thus attention to symptom management is of the utmost priority. Pain may be the consequence of rib or vertebral compression fractures which may occur as a result of osteoporosis (bone loss) that is associated with prolonged corticosteroid therapy. Treatment may be compromised by the limited pulmonary reserve. When tolerated, long-acting opioids can be used alone or in combination with non-steroidal anti-inflammatory drug (Hansen-Flaschen, 2000; Light et al., 1989). Mechanical supports are often recommended are often recommended for patients with compression fractures, but may be poorly tolerated in patients with COPD as they can constrain diaphragmatic excursion. (Lukert, 1994)

In caring for the terminally ill patient with little or no pulmonary reserve, it is more helpful to consider the therapeutic options in alleviating suffering than focus on the treatment of the disease. Lastly a thought should be given to withdrawal of life support if this is in line with the patients known wishes.

4.4. Hospice Care

Increasingly patients involved in the care of the dying advocate expanding access to hospice care for patients with COPD, heart failure and other chronic disease. However, to be eligible, these patients typically must have a projected survival of six months or less. According to the National Hospice and Palliative Care Organization's 2003 estimate, lung diseases as a whole accounted for 6.7% of hospice admissions and 6.8% of hospice deaths (The National Hospice and Palliative Care Organization, 2002; The National Hospice and Palliative Care Organization, 2005). The 2000 National Home and Hospice Care Survey estimated that 4.3% (4,500) of then current hospice patients had a primary diagnosis of COPD, and 5.5% (13,100) a secondary diagnosis. When hospice discharges are analyzed, COPD as a primary diagnosis accounts for 4.4% (27,600) of all hospice discharges, and 4.7% (38,000) when as a secondary diagnosis. The discharges for COPD diagnosis have been rising since 1996 (General Accounting Office, 2000; Haupt, 2003). Even though COPD is the fourth leading cause of death in the US it accounts for less than 5% of hospice cases.

Patients receiving hospice care have a greater variability in survival time compared to cancer patients. At least one study does show that there is a longer survival for COPD patients in hospice care compared to non-hospice care (Christakis and Escarce, 1996; Fox et al., 1999; Pyenson et al., 2004). The cost for hospice care compared to non hospice care is generally less, but when compared to cancer patients receiving hospice care is considerably higher given the different death trajectory (Gage and Dao, 2000; Pyenson et al., 2004). For example, Pyenson and associates conducted a cost comparison between patients who do or do not elect to receive Medicaid-paid hospice benefits. The study included data for 8,700 Medicare beneficiaries. For the majority of cohorts, mean and median Medicare costs were lower for patients enrolled in hospice care. The lower costs were associated with a longer time until death (Christakis and Lamont, 2000; Connors et al., 1996; Fox et al., 1999). Current Medicare hospice benefit guidelines for pulmonary diseases (including COPD) enrollment include the following

- Presence of chronic lung disease as documented by any of the below
  - Disabling dyspnea at rest, poorly responsive or unresponsive to bronchodilators, resulting in decreased functional capacity, e.g., bed to chair

existence, fatigue, and cough; documentation of FEV1, after bronchodilator _ 30% of predicted is objective evidence for disabling dyspnea, but is not necessary to obtain.

- Progression of end-stage pulmonary disease, as evidenced by increasing visits to the emergency department or hospitalizations for pulmonary infections and/or respiratory failure or increasing physician home visits prior to initial certification. Documentation of serial decrease of FEV1_ 40 mL/yr is objective evidence for disease progression, but is not necessary to obtain.

- Hypoxemia at rest on room air, as evidenced by Po2 _ 55 mm Hg or oxygen saturation _ 88% on supplemental oxygen determined either by arterial blood gas levels or oxygen saturation monitors (these values may be obtained from recent hospital records) or hypercapnia, as evidenced by Pco2 _ 50 mm Hg. This value may be obtained from recent (within 3 mo) hospital records.
- Right heart failure secondary to pulmonary disease (cor pulmonale), *e.g.*, not secondary to left heart disease or valvulopathy.
- Unintentional progressive weight loss of_ 10% of body weight over the preceding 6 mo.
- Resting tachycardia _ 100 beats/min.
- Documentation certifying terminal status must contain enough information to confirm terminal status upon review. Documentation meeting the above criteria would meet this requirement. If the patient does not meet the above criteria, yet is deemed appropriate for hospice care, sufficient documentation of the patient's condition that justifies terminal status, in the absence of meeting the above criteria, would be necessary. Documentation might include comorbidities, rapid decline in physical or functional status in spite of appropriate treatment, or symptom severity that with reasonable reliability is consistent with a life span prognosis of_ 6 mo.

In attempting to determine eligibility for hospice enrollment one should take into account several other factors aside from the Medicare guidelines above.

- Patients disease has progressed to the point that they may die because of any intercurrent illness, despite having been optimally treated,
- Age of patient: > 65 yrs
- Functional status of the patient as measured by various HRQOL instruments as well as the already utilized Karnofsky scale for general hospice care for malignant disease. That is patients are severely limited in their performance status.
- Number of admissions to hospital for AECOPD; a history of previous intubation during an AECOPD admission carrying with it a higher mortality
- Nutritional status and BMI
- The number of associated comorbidities, especially cardiac comorbidities such as ischemic heart disease and heart failure
- The patient understands that death may be near and does not wish to suffer needlessly

Recommending and electing for palliative care / hospice care in COPD is still studded with controversies including prognostication and cost benefits. Prognosticating as to which patient will survive for less than six months (as we have seen) has proven to be inaccurate. It is important to recognize that patients with COPD follow a dying trajectory different from those with cancer. Thus they may have prolonged courses prior to death in what is known as entry re-entry pattern. This pattern of uncertainty as well as the lack of ability to accurately predict mortality in COPD, should not exclude patients from the benefits of palliative and hospice care services. In fact the group of patients and their families may benefit more from palliative care enrollment from a psycho-social and spiritual standpoint. (Rabow et al., 2004) Frank discussions about patterns of dying and likely prognosis should be done in patients at risk.

The cost benefit of electing hospice care is still debated, since patients with COPD who elect hospice seem to live longer than patients with terminal cancer. This seems to be directly related to the length of hospice care. Although the expenditures are relatively higher compared to cancer patients the benefits may offset this. Patients in these programs either at home, in nursing homes, or in hospitals, are provided with comprehensive care to address their physical, emotional, spiritual and family needs. This in itself may prove to be a life prolonging measure while promoting all around increase in the quality of life.

5. Conclusion

In summary identifying the appropriate COPD patient who will benefit from a palliative care approach is to say the least challenging. None the less palliative therapy is a much underutilized path of therapy for this population. Prognostication of patients is still imperfect and there is a great need to have better models. Palliation for the COPD patient as well as other diseases with this reentry type of dying trajectory can become confusing for the family, patient and the physician. However by discussing the probabilities of various outcomes with the patient, identifying their preferences for measures such as intubation and other advance directives will help as guides. Emotional, spiritual and physical relief of symptoms should be the focus of the interventions offered by the palliative care team as opposed to only specific laboratory and physiologic measurements.

Glossary

Parenchyma: the functional parts of an organ such as the alveoli of the lungs (final portions of the respiratory tree which are involved in gas exchange), in contrast to the stroma which refers to the supporting tissues of organs.

Bronchodilator: an agent/ medication that reduces narrowing of the airways and obstruction of the airways in asthma and COPD.

FEV_1: The volume of gas exhaled during the first second of expiration.

FVC: The total volume of gas exhaled during expiration.

Hypercapnia: elevation of the carbon dioxide content of the blood above the upper limit of normal (the normal upper limit of carbon dioxide in arterial blood is 40mmHg) which may occur in respiratory insufficiency or hypoventilation.

Intubation: insertion of an endotracheal tube for the purpose of mechanical ventilation.

Pulmonary Embolism: an often fatal blood clot in the blood vessels of the lungs.

Cardiac Arrhythmia: an abnormality of the heart rhythm which is often accompanied by abnormality of the blood pressure or cardiac arrest.

Cor pulmonale: right sided heart failure secondary to pulmonary hypertension.

Opioid medications: narcotic medications such as morphine, oxycodone, fentanyl or hydromorphone which are most commonly used to treat pain but can also be used to relieve shortness of breath.

Vagotomy: surgical interruption of the vagus nerve.

Hypercarbic respiratory failure: respiratory failure that is accompanied by respiratory failure.

Albumin: a protein that is predominantly synthesized in the liver and maintains oncotic pressure and is reduced in cachexia, advanced medical illnesses and chronic liver disease. Normal values for serum albumin range from 3.5-5.5g/dl.

References

Almagro, P. (2002). Mortality after hospitalization for COPD (Consecutive admissions for AECOPD to a single teaching hospital). *Chest.* 121:1441-1448.

American Thoracic Society / European Respiratory Society. (2004). *Standards for the diagnosis and management of patients with COPD,* Copyrights 2004 American Thoracic Society and European Respiratory Society, available at http://www.thoracic.org/copd/pdf/copddoc.pdf, accessed December 2004.

Anthonisen, N.R., Connett, J.E., and Murray, R.P. for the Lung Health Study Research Group. (2002). Smoking and Lung Function of Lung Health Study Participants after 11 Years. *American Journal of Respiratory and Critical Care Medicine.* 166(5):675-679.

Anthonisen, N.R., Skeans, M.A., Wise, R.A., Manfreda, J., Kanner, R.E., and Connett, J.E. for the Lung Health Study Research Group. (2005). The Effects of a Smoking Cessation Intervention on 14.5-Year Mortality A Randomized Clinical Trial. *Annals of Internal Medicine.* 142(4):233-239.

Anthonisen, N.R. (1986). Prognosis in chronic obstructive pulmonary disease. *American Review of Respiratory Disease.* 133:14-20.

Argyropoulou, P., Patakas, D., Koukou, A., Vasiliadis, P., and Georgopoulos, D. (1993). Buspirone effect on breathlessness and exercise performance in patients with chronic obstructive pulmonary disease. *Respiration*. 60(4):216-220.

Barnes, P.J. (2000). Chronic obstructive pulmonary disease. *New England Journal of Medicine*. 343(4):269-80.

Benditt, J.O. (2000). Noninvasive ventilation at the end of life. *Respiratory Care*. 45: 1376-1381.

Berglund, E., Furhoff, A.K., Lofstrom B., and Oquist L. (1971). A study of the effects of unilateral vagus nerve block in a dyspnoeic patient. *Scandanavian Journal of Respiratory Disease*. 52 (1):34-38.

Booth, S., Anderson, H., Kite, S., Swannick, M., and Anderson, H. for the Expert Working Group of the Scientific Committee of the Association of Palliative Medicine. (2004). The use of oxygen in the palliation of breathlessness. A report of the expert working committee of the association of palliative medicine. *Scandanavian Journal of Respiratory Medicine*. 98:66-77.

Borg, G. (1990). Psychophysical scaling with applications in physical work and the perception of exertion, *Scandanavian Journal of Work and Environmental Health*.; 16 Suppl 1:55-8.

BTS guidelines for the management of chronic obstructive pulmonary disease. The COPD Guidelines Group of the Standards of Care Committee of the BTS. *Thorax*, 1997. 52 Suppl 5:S1-28.

Campbell, D.E., Lynn, J., Louis, T.A., and Shugarman L.R. (2004). Medicare program expenditures associated with hospice use. *Annals of Internal Medicine*. 140(4): 269-277.

Cazzolli, P.A. and Oppenheimer, E.A. (1996). Home mechanical ventilation for amyotrophic lateral sclerosis: nasal compared to tracheostomy-intermittent positive pressure ventilation. *Journal of the Neurological Sciences*. 139:123-128.

Celli, B.R., Cote, C.G., Marin, J.M., Casanova, C., Montes de Oca, M., Mendez, R.A., Pinto Plata, V., and Carbal, H.J. (2004). The body-mass index, airflow obstruction, dyspnea and exercise capacity index in chronic obstructive pulmonary disease. *New England Journal of Medicine*. 350(10):1005-1011.

Chailleux, E., Laaban, J.P., and Veale, D. (2003) Prognostic value of nutritional depletion in patients with COPD treated by long-term oxygen therapy. *Chest*. 123 (5):1460-1466.

Cherny, N.I. and Portenoy, R.K. (1994). Sedation in the management of refractory symptoms: guidelines for evaluation and treatment. *Journal of Palliative Care*. 10(2):31-8.

Christakis, N.A. and Escarce, J.J. (1996). Survival of Medicare patients after enrollment in hospice programs. *New England Journal of Medicine*. 335(3):172-178.

Christakis, N.A. and Lamont, E.B. (2000). Extent and determinants of error in doctors prognosis in terminally ill patients: prospective cohort study. *British Medical Journal*. 320 (7233):469-472.

Claessens, M.T., Lynn, J., Zhong, Z., Desbiens, N.A., Phillips, R.S., Wu, A.W., Harrell, F.E., and Connors, A.F. (2000). Dying with lung cancer or chronic obstructive pulmonary disease: insights from SUPPORT. Study to Understand Prognoses and Preferences for Outcomes and Risks of Treatments. *Journal of the American Geriatric Society*. 48 (suppl. 5):S146-153.

Connors, A.F., Dawson, N.V., Thomas, C., Harrell, F.E., Desbiens, N.A., Fulkerson, W.J., Bellamy, P., Goldman, L., and Knaus, W.A. (1996). Outcomes following acute exacerbation of severe chronic obstructive lung disease. The SUPPORT investigators (Study to Understand Prognoses and Preferences for Outcomes and

Risks of Treatments). *American Journal of Respiratory and Critical Care Medicine.* 154(4 Pt 1):959-67.

Continuous or nocturnal oxygen therapy in hypoxemic chronic obstructive lung disease: a clinical trial. Nocturnal Oxygen Therapy Trial Group. (1980). *Annals of Internal Medicine.* 93(3):391-8.

Costello, R., Deegan, P., Fitzpatrick, M., and McNicholas, W.T. (1997). Reversible hypercapnia in chronic obstructive pulmonary disease: A distinct pattern of respiratory failure with a favorable prognosis. *American Journal of Medicine.* 103:239.

Current estimates from the National Health Interview Survey, 1995. Vital and health statistics. (1996). Centers for Disease Control and Prevention: Washington, D.C.

Decramer, M., Gosselink, R., Troosters, T., Verschueren, M., and Evers, G. (1997). Muscle weakness is related to utilization of health care resources in COPD patients. *European Respiratory Journal.* 10(2):417-423.

Dolan, S. and Varkey, B. (2005). Prognostic factors in chronic obstructive pulmonary disease. *Current Opinions in Pulmonary Medicine.* 11(2):149-152.

Domingo-Salvany, A., Lamarca, R., Ferrer, M., and Garcia-Aymerich J. (2002). Health-related quality of life and mortality in male patients with Chronic Obstructive Pulmonary Disease. *American Journal of Respiratory and Critical Care Medicine.* 166(5):680-685.

Dyspnea. (1999). Mechanisms, assessment, and management: a consensus statement. American Thoracic Society. *American Journal of Respiratory and Critical Care Medicine.* 159(1):321-40.

Edmonds, P., Karlsen, S., Khan, S., and Addington-Hall, J. (2001). A comparison of the palliative care needs of patients dying from chronic respiratory diseases and lung cancer. *Palliative Medicine.* 15(4):287-95.

Elkington H., White P., Addington-Hall J., Higgs R., and Edmonds P. The healthcare needs of chronic obstructive pulmonary disease patients in the last year of life. *Palliative Medicine.* 2005 Sep; 19(6):485-491.

Elliott, M.W., Simonds, A.K., Carroll, M.P., Wedzicha, J.A., and Branthwaite, M.A. (1992). Domiciliary nocturnal nasal intermittent positive pressure ventilation in hypercapnic respiratory failure due to chronic obstructive lung disease: effects on sleep and quality of life. *Thorax.* 47(5):342-348.

Fagon, J.Y., and Chastre, J. (1996). Severe exacerbations of COPD patients: the role of pulmonary infections. *Seminars in Respiratory Infections.* 11(2):109-118.

Fan, V.S., Curtis, J.R., Tu, S.P., McDonell M.B., and Fihn, S.D., for the Ambulatory Care Quality Improvement Project Investigators. (2002). Using Quality of Life to Predict Hospitalization and Mortality in Patients With Obstructive Lung Diseases. *Chest.* 122(2):429-436.

Ferrer, M., Alonso, J., Morera, J., Marrades, R.M., Khalaf, A., Aguar, M.C., Plaza, V., Prieto, and Anto, J.M. (1997). Chronic obstructive pulmonary disease stage and health-related quality of life. *Annals of Internal Medicine.* 127(12):1072-1079.

Fletcher, C. and Peto, R. (1977). The natural history of chronic airflow obstruction. *British Medical Journal.* 1977. 1(6077):1645-8.

Fox, E., Landrum-Mcniff, K., Dawson, N.V., Wu, A.W., Zhong Z., and Lynn, J. (1999). Evaluation of prognositic criteria for determining hospice eligibility in patients with advanced lung, heart, or liver disease. *Journal of the American Medical Association.* 282(17):1638-1645.

Gage, B., Dao, T. Medicare's Hospice Benefit: Use and Expenditures. March 2000 Report to US Department of Health and Human Services. Available at http://aspe.os.dhhs.gov/daltcp/reports/96useexp.htm#section3b

General Accounting Office. September 2000. Medicare: More Beneficiaries Use Hospice but for Fewer Days of Care. Publication no. GAO:HEHS-00-182 Washington DC: General Accounting Office, 2000.

Goel, A., Pinckney, R.G., and Littenberg, B. (2003). APACHE II predicts long-term survival in COPD patients admitted to a general medical ward. *Journal of General Internal Medicine.* 18(10):824-830.

Groenewegen, K.H., Schols, A.M.W.J., and Wouters E.F.M. (2003). Mortality and mortality related factors after hospitalization for acute exacerbation of COPD. *Chest.* 124:459-467.

Guyatt, G.H., Feeny, D.H., and Patrick, D.L. (1993). Measuring heath-related quality of life. *Annals of Internal Medicine.* 118:622-629.

Hajiro, T., Nishimura, K., Tsukino, M., Ikeda, A., Koyama, H., and Izumi, T. (1998). Comparison of discriminative properties among disease-specific questionnaires for measuring health-related quality of life in patients with chronic obstructive pulmonary disease. *American Journal of Respiratory and Critical Care Medicine.* 157(3 Pt 1):785-790.

Halpern, M.T., Stanford, R.H, and Borker, R. (2003). The burden of COPD in the U.S.A.: results from the Confronting COPD survey. *Respiratory Medicine.* 97 Suppl 3: p. S81-9.

Hansell, J.A. Walk, J.B. Soriano, and A.L. (2003). What do chronic obstructive pulmonary disease patients die from? A multiple cause coding analysis; *European Respiratory Journal.* 22: 809-814.

Hansen-Flaschen, J.H. (2000). Palliative home care for advanced lung disease. *Respiratory Care* 45:1478-1486; discussion 1486-1479.

Haupt, B.J. Vital and Health Statistics; Characteristics of Hospice Care Discharges and their length of service: United States, 2000. National Center for Health Statistics. Vital Health Stat 13(154):1-36. Available at http://www.cdc.gov/nchs/data/series/sr_13/sr13_154.pdf

Heffner, J.E., Fahy, B., Hilling, L., and Barbieri, C. (1996). Attitudes regarding advance directives among patients in pulmonary rehabilitation. *American Journal of Respiratory and Critical Care Medicine.* 154(6Pt 1):1735-1740.

Heffner, J.E. (2000). Role of pulmonary rehabilitation in palliative care. *Respiratory Care.* 45(11):1365-1371; discussion 1371-1365.

Hilleman, D.E., Dewan, N., Malesker, M., and Friedman, M. (2000). Pharma coeconomic evaluation of COPD. *Chest.* 118(5):1278-1285.

Howard, P., Gorzelak, K., Lahdensuo, A., Strom, K., Tobiasz, M., and Weitzenbaum, E. (1997). Causes of death in patients with COPD and chronic respiratory failure. *Monaldi Archives for Chest Disease.* 52(1):43-47.

Hurd, S.S. (2000). International efforts directed at attacking the problem of COPD. *Chest.* 117(5 Suppl 2): p. 336S-8S.

James, A.L., Palmer, L.J., Kicic, E., Maxwell, P.S., Lagan, S.E., Ryan, G.F., and Musk, A.W. (2005). Decline in lung function in the Busselton Health Study: the effects of asthma and cigarette smoking. *American Journal of Respiratory and Critical Care Medicine.* 171(2):109-114.

James L. and Hallenbeck M. Palliative Care Perspectives: Oxford University Press, Inc., 2003.

Jennings, A.L., Davies, A.N., Higgins, J.P., Gibbs, J.S., and Broadley, K.E. (2002). A systematic review of the use of opiods in the management of dyspnea, *Thorax.* 57(11):939-944

Jobst, K., Chen, J.H., McPherson, K., Arrowsmith, T., Brown, V., Effthimiou, J., Fletcher, H.J., Maciocia, G., Mole, P., and Shifrin, K. (1986). Controlled trial of acupuncture for disabling breathlessness. Lancet. 2(8521-22):1416-1419.

Kessler, R., Faller, M., Fourgaut, G., Mennecier, B., and Weitzenblum, E. (1999). Predictive factors of hospitalization for acute exacerbation in a series of 64 patients with chronic obstructive pulmonary disease. *American Journal of Respiratory and Critical Care Medicine.* 159 (1):158-164.

Knaus, W.A., Harrell, F.E., Lynn, J., Goldman L., Phillips, R.S., Connors, A.F., Dawson, N.V., Fulkerson, W.J., Califf, R.M., Desbiens, N., Layde, P., Oye, R.K., Bellamy, P.E., Hakim, R.B., and Wagner, D.P. (1995). The SUPPORT prognostic Model. Objective estimates of survival for seriously ill hospitalized adults. *Annals of Internal Medicine.* 122(3):191-203.

Light, R.W., Merrill, E.J., Despars, J.A., Gordon, G.H., and Mutalipassi, L.R. (1985). Prevalence of depression and anxiety in patients with COPD. Relationship to functional capacity. *Chest.* 87(1):35-38

Light, R.W., Muro, J.R., Sato, R.I., Stansbury, D.W., Fischer, C.E., and Brown, S.E. (1989). Effects of oral morphine on breathlessness and exercise tolerance in patients with chronic obstructive pulmonary disease. *The American Review of Respiratory Disease.* 139(1):126-133.

Lopez, A.D. and Murray, C.C. (1998). The global burden of disease, 1990-2020. Nat Med. 4(11):1241-3.

Lukert, B.P. (1994). Vertebral compression fractures: how to manage pain, avoid disability. *Geriatrics.* 49(2):22-26.

Lunney, J.R., Lynn, J., Foley, D., Lipson, S., and Guralnik, J.M. (2003). Patterns of functional decline at the end of life. *Journal of the American Medical Association.* 289(18):2387-2392.

Lynn, J., Ely, E.W., Zhong, Z., McNiff, K.L., Dawson, N.V., Connors, A., Desbiens, N.A., Classens, M., and McCarthy, E.P. (2000). Living and dying with COPD. *Journal of the American Geriatric Society.* 48(5 Suppl):S91-S100.

Maa, S.H., Gauthier, D., and Turner, M. (1997). Acupressure as an adjunct to a pulmonary rehabilitation program. *Journal of Cardiopulmonary Rehabilitation.* 17(4):268-276.

Mahler, D.A., Faryniarz, K., Tomlinson, D., Colice, G.L., Robbins, A.G., Olmstead, E.M., and O'Connor, G.T. (1992). Impact of dyspnea and physiologic function on general health status in patients with chronic obstructive pulmonary disease. *Chest.* 102 (2):395-401.

Mahler D.A. (2000). How Should Health-Related Quality of Life Be Assessed in Patients With COPD?. *Chest* 117:54S-57S.

Mahler, D.A. and Mackowiak, J.I. (1995). Evaluation of the Short-Form 36-item questionnaire to measure health-related quality of life in patients with COPD. *Chest* 107 (Suppl 2):1585-1589

Manning, H.L. (2000). Dyspnea treatment. *Respiratory Care.* 45:1342-1350.

Mannino, D., Gagnon, R.C., Petty, T.L., and Lydick, E. (2000). Obstructive lung disease and low lung function in adults in the United States: Data from the National Health and Nutrition Examination Survey, 1988-1994; *Archives of Internal Medicine.* 160(11):1683-89.

Mannino, D.M. (2002). COPD: Epidemiology, prevalence, morbidity and mortality, and heterogeneity; *Chest* 121 (suppl 5):121S-126S.

Mannino, D.M., Homa, D.M., Akinbami, L.J., Ford, E.S., and Redd, S.C. (2002). Chronic Obstructive Pulmonary Disease Surveillance — United States, 1971–2000. *Morbidity and Mortality Weekly Report.* 51(6):1-16.

Mannino, D.M., Buist, A.S., Petty, T.L., Enright, P.L., and Redd, S.C. (2003) Lung function and mortality in the United States: data from the First National Health and Nutrition Examination Survey follow up study. *Thorax.,* 58(5):388-93.

Meyer, P.A., Mannino, D.M., Redd, S.C., and Olson, D.R. (2002). Characteristics of Adults Dying With COPD; *Chest.* 122(6):2003–2008.

Mitchell-Heggs, P., Murphy, K., Minty, K., Guz, A., Patterson, S.C., Minty, P.S. and Rosser, R.M. (1980). Diazepam in the treatment of dyspnoea in the 'Pink Puffer' syndrome. *The Quarterly Journal of Medicine.* 49(193):9-20.

Morbidity and Mortality: 2002 Chart Book on Cardiovascular, Lung and Blood Diseases., National Institutes of Health. National Heart, Lung and Blood Institute.

Murray, C.J. and Lopez, A.D. (1997). Alternative projections of mortality and disability by cause 1990-2020: Global Burden of Disease Study. *Lancet.* 349(9064): 498-504.

National Center for Health Statistics. Raw data from the National Health Interview Survey, U.S., 2002

Nevins, M.L. and Epstein, S.K. (2001). Predictors of outcome for patients with COPD requiring invasive mechanical ventilation. *Chest.* 119(6):1840-1849.

Nocturnal Oxygen Therapy Trial Group. (1980). Continuous or nocturnal oxygen therapy in hypoxemic chronic obstructive lung disease. *Annals of Internal Medicine.* 93(3):391-398.

Osman, L.M., Godden, D.J., and Friend, J.A.R. (1997). Quality of life and hospital re-admission in patients with chronic obstructive pulmonary disease. *Thorax* 52:67-71.

Patil, S.P., Krishnan, J.A., Lechtzin, N., and Dietze, G.B. (2003). In-hospital mortality following acute exacerbations of chronic obstructive pulmonary disease. *Archives of Internal Medicine.* 163(10):1180-1186.

Pauwels, R.A., Buist, A.S., and Calverley, P.M., for the GOLD Scientific Committee. Global strategy for the diagnosis, management, and prevention of chronic obstructive pulmonary disease, 2004 Update. NHLBI/WHO Global Initiative for Chronic Obstructive Lung Disease (GOLD) Workshop summary. Available at www.gold-copd.com accessed December 2004.

Perrin, C., El Far, Y., Vandenbos, F., Tamisier, R., Dumon, M.C., Lemoigne, F., Mouroux, J., and Blaive, B. (1997). Domiciliary nasal intermittent positive pressure ventilation in severe COPD: effects on lung function and quality of life. *European Respiratory Journal.* 10(12):2835-2839.

Pyenson, B., Connor, S., Fitch, K., and Kinzbrunner, B. (2004). Medicare cost in matched hospice and non-hospice cohorts. *Journal of Pain and Symptom Management.* 28(3):200-210.

Rabow, M.W., Dibble, S.L., Pantilat, S.Z., and McPhee, S.J. (2004). The comprehensive care team: a controlled trial of outpatient palliative medicine consulation. *Archives of Internal Medicine.* 164(1):83-91.

Santo Tomas, L.H. and Varkey, B. (2004). Improving health-related quality of life in COPD. *Current Opinion in Pulmonary Medicine.* 10(2):120-127.

Seneff, M.G., Wagner, D.P., Wagner, R.P., Zimmerman, J.E., and Knaus, W.A. (1995). Hospital and 1-year survival of patients admitted to intensive care units with acute exacerbation of chronic obstructive pulmonary disease. *Journal of the American Medical Association.* 274(23):1852-57.

Siafakas, N.M., Vermiere, P., Pride, N.B., Paoletti, P., Gibson, J., Howard, P., Yernault, J.C., Descramer, M., Higenbottam, T., and Postma, D.S. (1995). Optimal assessment and management of chronic obstructive pulmonary disease (COPD). The European Respiratory Society Task Force. *European Respiratory Journal.* 8(8):1398-420.

Sibuya, M., Yamada, M., Kanamaru, A., Tanaka, K., Suzuki, H., Noguchi, E., Altose, M.D., and Homma, I. (1994). Effect of chest wall vibration on dyspnea in patients with chronic respiratory disease. *American Journal of Respiratory and Critical Care Medicine.* 149(5):1235-40.

Sin, D.D., Stafinski, T., Ng, Y.C., Bell, N.R., and Jacobs, P. (2002). The impact of chronic obstructive pulmonary disease on work loss in the United States. *American Journal of Respiratory and Critical Care Medicine.* 165(5):704-7.

Smoller, J.W., Pollack, M.H., Systrom, D., and Kradin, R.L. (1998). Sertraline effects on dyspnea in patients with obstructive airways disease. *Psychosomatics* 39(1):24-29.

Sorenson, H.M. (2000).Dyspnea assessment. *Respiratory Care.* 45(11):1331-1338.

Spence, D.P., Graham, D.R., Ahmed, J. Rees, K., Pearson, M.G., and Calverley, P.M. (1993). Does cold air affect exercise capacity and dyspnea in stable chronic obstructive pulmonary disease? *Chest.* 103(3):693-696.

Standards for the diagnosis and care of patients with chronic obstructive pulmonary disease. American Thoracic Society. *American Journal of Respiratory and Critical Care Medicine.* 1995. 152(5 Pt 2):S77-121.

Strassels, S.A., Smith D.H., Sullivan, S.D., and Mahajan, P.S. (2001). The costs of treating COPD in the United States. *Chest,* 2001. 119(2):344-52.

Strumpf, D.A., Millman, R.P., Carlisle, C.C., Grattan Ryan, S.M., Erickson, A.D., and Hill, N.S. (1991). Nocturnal positive pressure ventilation via nasal mask in patients with severe COPD. *The American Review of Respiratory Disease.* 144(6):1234-1239.

Sullivan, S.D., Ramsey, S.D., and Lee, T.A. (2000). The economic burden of COPD. Chest. 117(2 Suppl): p. 5S-9S.

Sutherland, E.R. and Cherniack R.M. (2004). Management of chronic obstructive pulmonary disease. *The New England Journal of Medicine.* 350(26):2689-97.

The National Hospice and Palliative Care Organization's 2002 National Data Set Summary Report, available at http://www.nhpco.org/files/members/2002National DataSet.pdf, accessed January 2005.

The National Hospice and Palliative Care Organization's Facts and Figures on Hospice, available at http://www.nhpco.org/files/public/Hospice_Facts_110104.pdf, accessed on January 2005.

Teno, J.M., Weitzen, S., Fennell, M.L., and Mor, V. (2001). Dying trajectory in the last year of life: does cancer trajectory fit other diseases? *Journal of Palliative Medicine.* 4(4):457-64

Testa, M.A., and Simonson, D.C. (1996). Assessment of quality-of-life outcomes. *New England Journal of Medicine.* 334(13):835-840.

Yach, D., Hawkes, C., Gould, C.L., and Hofman, K.J. (2004). The global burden of chronic diseases overcoming impediments to prevention and control. *Journal of American Medical Association.* 291(21):2616-2622.

Zielinski, J., MacNee, W., Wedzicha, J., Ambrosino, N., Braghiroli, A., and Dolensky, J. (1997). Causes of death in patients with COPD and chronic respiratory failure. *The Monaldi Archives of Chest Disease.* 52:43-47.

8
Palliative Care and Chronic Heart Failure

Vikas Bhatara MD, Edmund H. Sonnenblick MD,
Thierry H. Le Jemtel MD, and Vladimir Kvetan MD

1. Introduction

Congestive heart failure is a serious and ultimately fatal illness, and there is currently no cure except for cardiac transplantation. Congestive heart failure (CHF) is a leading cause of morbidity and mortality. It is associated with marked impairments in health related quality of life, emotional and physical wellbeing. It is a leading cause of admission to acute care hospitals and subsequent readmission. Despite the high prevalence and high physical and psychosocial burden patients with CHF are underserved by palliative care and hospice programs. In this chapter we will describe the pathophysiological processes that underlie the functional complications of congestive heart failure, describe the natural history of congestive heart failure, the modes of demise of patients with CHF, its major subcategories: diastolic and systolic dysfunction. We will make recommendations for appropriate timing of referral to palliative care and hospice and describe the potential benefits for the inclusion of palliative care teams in the provision of care to patients with CHF and their families.

2. Epidemiology

As prevalence increases, nearly five million in the U.S. population are burdened by congestive heart failure and 500,000 new cases are diagnosed each year. In 2001, approximately 53,000 patients died of CHF as the primary cause, 264,000 died of CHF as a secondary cause, and the death toll is still rising. Overall mortality continues at 50% within five years after diagnosis.

VIKAS BHATARA • Critical Care Medicine, Montefiore Medical Center of the Albert Einstein College of Medicine, 111th East 210th Street, Bronx, NY 10467.   EDMUND H. SONNENBLICK • Cardiology, Jack D. Weiler Hospital of the Albert Einstein College of Medicine, 1825 Eastchester Road, Bronx, NY 10461.   THIERRY H. Le JEMTEL • Tulane University School of Medicine, Section of Cardiology, 1430 Tulane Avenue, SL 48, New Orleans, LA 70112.   VLADIMIR KVETAN • Critical Care Medicine, Montefiore Medical Center of the Albert Einstein College of Medicine, 111th East 210th Street, Bronx, NY 10467.

But mortality also depends on the degree of symptoms and functional impairment. Once a patient has symptoms with no exertion (New York Heart Association class 1), the mortality rate is as high as 60% at 12 months. For patients with no symptoms at any level of exertion (NYHA class I) mortality is in the 10% range at 12 months.

CHF is largely a disease of the elderly. Starting at age 55, 6% of men have CHF and this increases to 10% at age 75 and over. In women 2% have CHF at age 55 and this increases to 10.9% at 75 and over. CHF is the major reason for emergent hospitalization in individuals over 65 and a frequent source of readmission, with about 80% of rehospitalizations for CHF occurring in the over-65 population. CHF is the most costly cardiovascular illness. In 2005, the total direct and indirect costs were estimated at $27.9 billion; approximately $2.9 billion annually is spent on drugs for treatment. Estimated costs increased to $29.6 billion in 2006. The hospitalization costs alone for CHF exceed those of all myocardial infarctions (MI, heart attacks) and cancers combined. The hospitalization costs alone for CHF exceed those of all myocardial infarctions and cancers combined. In 1997 an estimated $5501 was spent for every hospital discharge diagnosis of heart failure and an additional $1742 was required per month to care for patients after hospital discharge. (Garg et al., 1993; American Heart Association, 1998; American Heart Association, 2000; Graves, 1990; O'Connell and Bristow, 1994; AHA, ACC Guidelines Update, 2005; McAlister et al., 1999; Stevenson, 2001).

CHF is not only incurable but the pain and suffering can be considerable. Of patients dying of CHF, 60% have severe breathing problems. Pain occurs in up to 78% of patients dying with advanced heart disease. Among seriously ill hospitalized patients with congestive heart failure 41% experienced moderate to severe pain in the last 3 days of life. Up to 40% of patients have impaired ability to communicate and 20% were not conscious in the three days prior to death. Other common physical symptoms include anorexia and fatigue. More than one-third of hospitalized CHF patients are reported to suffer from major depression and depression in CHF patients appears to be associated with increased risk for mortality and rehospitalization (McCarthy et al., 1996; Levenson et al., 2000; SUPPORT, 1995; Lynn et al., 1997; Koenig, 1997; Jiang et al., 2001).

Exacerbations and repeated hospitalizations are frequent in heart failure. At 24 hours before death, patients with advanced heart failure were predicted to have an 80% chance of being alive in two months time. Other patients were predicted to have a greater than 50% chance of surviving for six months, but died within three days. These were key findings in the SUPPORT trial; predictions were made during a first hospitalization for heart failure (Study to Understand Prognoses and Risks of Treatment). The trajectory of frequent crises with return almost to a prior baseline level of functioning and then a gradual functional decline makes identification of individual patients who are actively dying difficult. The lack of a pronounced decline in functional status in contrast to that seen in cancer in the last months of life may account for some of the delays in referral to hospice and underutilization of the

Medicare hospice benefit for patients with CHF. Only about 10% of patients who enroll in hospice do so with CHF as the hospice diagnosis. Lengths of stay on hospice are typically brief. This limits the ability to provide clinical benefit to patients and their families and may lessen the cost savings that result from reduced hospitalization (SUPPORT, 1995; Pyenson *et al.*, 2004).

Patients with end-stage organ failure are often not referred to palliative care services because there is not a readily identifiable terminal phase of illness. In a British study, Hanratty and associates at the University of Liverpool set up focus groups with primary care physicians and specialists in cardiology, geriatrics and palliative medicine to explore views about palliative care for patients with heart failure. Participants were reluctant to endorse expansion of specialized palliative care in this setting. An unpredictable course of heart failure was cited as one of the barriers to developing approaches to palliative care.

Another study by Murray and associates, University of Edinburgh, compared patients with inoperable lung cancer and those with advanced CHF. Patients with CHF had less information and understanding about their illness and its progression, were more limited in decision-making and in access to palliative care services. Again this study confirmed that predicting illness trajectory is much more difficult in advanced heart failure than in cancer. There is a high degree of uncertainty, potentially preventing physicians from identifying patients who have reached the terminal phase of illness and implementing palliative care (Hanratty *et al.*, 2002; Murray *et al.*, 2002).

3. The Pathophysiology of Congestive Heart Failure

From a physiological standpoint, the failure of the cardiac pump to adequately meet the metabolic requirements of the body, especially during physical activity, defines chronic heart failure. From a clinical standpoint, CHF is not a primary disease but a syndrome that is the end result of many cardiac and vascular diseases. If systemic hypertension, coronary artery disease and diabetes mellitus were to be either prevented or more adequately treated, the syndrome of CHF would not have reached epidemic proportions and the issue of the provision and the timing of palliative care for patients with CHF would concern far fewer patients Albert 2002. Thus, the syndrome of CHF commonly develops largely when the therapy aimed at the primary culprit disease has failed. When either hypertension is well controlled or obstructive coronary artery disease stabilized so that no further myocardium is lost, left ventricular (LV) function may remain chronically reduced but chronic heart failure may not ensue. However, when LV dysfunction is allowed to progress or its progression cannot be stopped, a decline in LV performance eventually compromises kidney function, and promotes skeletal muscle atrophy, systemic inflammation and catabolism, the destructive phase of metabolism. Despite markedly reduced LV systolic performance functional capacity as assessed with the NYHA classification model or determination of peak aerobic capacity may remain normal for relatively long periods of time. However, once progression of LV dysfunction has led to peripheral manifestations of limited cardiac output, functional capacity steadily decreases. The peripheral manifestation of heart failure can include an increase in dyspnea, fatigue, reduced exercise capacity, fluid retention or swelling. Respiratory complaints include dyspnea when lying flat, cough and wheezing, paroxysmal episodes of dyspnea. Abdominal symptoms can include bloating, early satiety, weight gain, right upper quadrant pain, also loss of appetite, weight loss, nausea and vomiting. Therapeutic intervention such as diuretics and unloading agents may stabilize or slow this process. What precisely triggers the onset of progressive CHF is still poorly understood but likely to be related to the inability to maintain preferential distribution of a limited cardiac output to essential organs. The loss of adequate peripheral blood flow distribution and its irreversibility account for the unavoidable poor outcome of patients with advanced CHF.

4. Classification of Heart Failure

The syndrome of CHF can be conveniently ascribed to predominantly left ventricular (LV) systolic dysfunction when the LV ejection fraction (fraction of blood pumped out of the ventricle with each beat) is below or equal to 40%. The major clinical manifestations of systolic dysfunction relate to an inadequate cardiac output, with weakness, fatigue, reduced exercise capacity and other symptoms of reduced blood flow. However symptoms of CHF may arise with no systolic abnormality; the LV ejection fraction is greater or equal to 50%. With diastolic LV dysfunction, the ventricle contracts normally but its walls have impaired relaxation and increased stiffness, so that less blood enters during normal filling. As a consequence blood backs up in the left atria and lung vessels and cause pulmonary congestion.

When LVEF is greater than 40% and lower than 50%, CHF is more likely due to a mix of LV systolic and diastolic dysfunction. Systolic ventricular dysfunction predominantly affects men 60 to 65 years of age and coronary artery disease is the most common primary disease. Diastolic ventricular dysfunction, which affects 20-50% of all CHF patients, commonly affects women 70 to 75 years of age and hypertension, diabetes and obesity are the common culprit conditions (Kitzman et al., 2002). Both systolic and diastolic ventricular dysfunction produce the same clinical syndrome of CHF although therapy and mortality rates differ. The mechanisms that are responsible for progression of systolic CHF are better understood than those responsible for progression of diastolic heart failure.

4.1. Addressing Systolic Ventricular Dysfunction

Acute loss of myocardium, the muscular layer of the ventricular wall, during a myocardial infarction, likewise chronic volume or pressure overload with valvular heart disease, trigger a sequence of events that are initially an adaptive response to protect the failing heart. Principally there is a change in architecture of the left ventricle, such that the chamber becomes a dilated, globular structure. Loss of myocytes, the cardiac muscle cells, is encountered by an increase in growth and size of the remaining myocytes, with a corresponding increase in thickness of the ventricular wall. These changes are referred to as myocardial or ventricular hypertrophy, respectively. All are part of the process of remodeling of the left ventricle to maintain cardiac pumping ability and cardiac output. Systolic overloading (hypertension) also leads to progressive LV remodeling with thickening of the LV wall, but initially without LV dilatation. With time and increasing failure of the myocardium due to hypertrophy, ventricular dilatation ensues. In the absence of co-morbid events, such as angina, LV remodeling and the gradual deterioration of LV systolic function remain clinically silent (Fig. 8.1). Symptoms of fatigue and shortness of breath during physical activity tend to be mild and loosely related to the extent of LV systolic dysfunction. For example average LVEF was 28% in the so called asymptomatic patients who were enrolled in the prevention arm of the Study Of Left Ventricular Dysfunction (SOLVD) trial of the role of enalapril in heart failure. The LVEF was only further reduced to 24 % in the symptomatic patients (as defined by the need for therapy) who were enrolled in the treatment arm of the trial. Thus, LV remodeling may be far advanced when symptoms of CHF first require attention. Symptoms of fatigue and shortness of breath may vary from patient to patient. They are most noticeable during physical activity and related to fluid accumulation. Moreover, these symptoms of increasing CHF become manifest from changes in the peripheral circulation and need no additional myocardial damage beyond what is already present. (The SOLVD investigators, 1992).

4.1.1. Treatment of Heart Failure

An important target of therapy is to slow, avert or somehow reverse remodeling. Beta-adrenergic blocking agents, angiotensin converting enzyme (ACE) inhibitors, and angiotensin receptor blockers are effective in attenuating the remodeling process. Beta-adrenergic blockers are the only agents proven experimentally to reverse remodeling. Cardiac failure is accompanied by compensatory mechanisms; one is vasoconstriction, a narrowing of blood vessels. In therapy, vasodilator drugs increase blood flow particularly in smaller arteries and arterioles, opposing the excessive vasoconstriction. Patients with LV failure who have low cardiac output and high filling pressures often benefit when elevated resistance is reduced by vasodilator therapy. Endothelial dysfunction in CHF can be improved with the use of ACE inhibitors for vasodilation. There is some evidence to suggest that the lipid-lowering statin drugs can also be beneficial; they modulate nitric oxide levels in vascular endothelium and thereby reduce platelet activation in experimental CHF models.

The factors that determine reversibility of the LV remodeling process in patients with CHF due to LV systolic dysfunction are incompletely understood. The duration and extent of systolic dysfunction appear to be important. In patients with dilated cardiomyopathy, the amount of myocardial fibrosis on right ventricular biopsy may be indicative of the extent of damage and when substantial suggests less potential for reversal of LV remodeling by long-term beta-adrenergic blockade. In contrast a higher systemic blood pressure indicates that patients with LV systolic dysfunction will experience a substantial anti-remodeling effect of long-term beta-adrenergic-blockade (Devereaux et al., 2004). The determinants of reversibility of the peripheral manifestations of CHF have not been formally investigated. Peripheral manifestations of CHF tend to be poorly reversible in patients with marked cachexia. The limited improvement of functional capacity after cardiac transplantation also underscores the lack of or partial reversibility of peripheral manifestations in patients with advanced CHF. Thus, close monitoring of functional capacity helps to optimize the time of referral to a palliative care program in patients with CHF due to LV systolic dysfunction. Referral to a palliative care program should be pursued when patients become home bound due to poor functional capacity.

4.2. Diastolic Ventricular Dysfunction

The mechanisms responsible for diastolic ventricular dysfunction and the time course of its progression vary substantially and are often obscure. In general, it is characterized by an increased LV diastolic pressure in the presence of a preserved ejection fraction. Thus, there is relative stiffening of the LV wall. This often occurs in the context of myocardial hypertrophy secondary to hypertension. The loss of cardiac myocytes with age especially in men also results in hypertrophy of the remaining myocytes and alters LV compliance. In women, systemic hypertension is the overwhelming pathological cause of ventricular diastolic dysfunction. Left ventricular mass is increased in 80% of patients with diastolic heart failure and a reduction in LV mass with treatment of hypertension is clearly associated with a better outcome (Devereaux et al., 2004). However the rate of progression of alteration in LV mass and the contribution of altered LV mass to reduced functional capacity are unclear in patients with diastolic heart failure. Similar to systolic heart failure, cardiac parameters such as indices of LV diastolic function and LV mass do not correlate with functional capacity in patients with diastolic heart failure. Functional capacity when evaluated by peak aerobic capacity is reduced to the same extent in patients with systolic and diastolic heart failure (Kaminsky et al., 2000). With diastolic dysfunction, cardiac output is limited by an increased heart rate, which limits time for diastolic ventricular filling. Thus, as with systolic heart failure, cardiac output becomes central to the development of CHF. As occurs in patients with systolic heart failure, peripheral manifestations are likely to contribute to reduced functional capacity in patients with diastolic heart failure. However in contrast to patients with systolic heart failure, alterations in skeletal muscle mass, metabolism and the proportion of different types of myocytes have not yet been reported in patients with diastolic heart failure.

4.3. Inexorable Progression of Heart Failure Despite Therapy

Although several factors can accelerate the process of cardiac remodeling, there is substantial evidence that activation of a number of neurohumeral systems plays an important role in remodeling, and thereby in the progression of CHF. For example, there is activation of the adrenergic nerve fibers of the sympathetic nervous system. Enhanced and sustained cardiac adrenergic drive occurs in heart failure and contributes to the progression of LV dysfunction and remodeling. The release of norepinephrine, the primary neurotransmitter, can exert a damaging effect on the myocytes and thus contributes to over stimulation of the remodeling process with progressive chamber dilatation and loss of contractile function.

Activation of the renin-angiotensin system in heart failure in response to low blood volume results in an increase in blood pressure and other adverse effects. Sympathetic activation accompanying heart failure also augments the release of renin and angiotensin II; among the effects is exaggerated increase in vascular and myocardial cell growth that again contributes to remodeling. A low serum sodium concentration (hyponatremia), which is inversely proportional to renin levels, has consistently predicted an unfavorable outcome (See Figure 8.1).

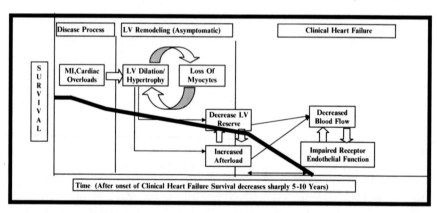

FIGURE 8.1. The syndrome of chronic heart failure is the end result of cardiac or vascular diseases that result from a loss of cardiac myocytes or long term exposure of the heart to volume or pressure overload. Once the syndrome is set off, it evolves in two stages: the left ventricle first undergoes remodeling and patients then develop peripheral manifestations leading to end-organ dysfunction. Left ventricular remodeling is clinically silent save for flare ups of co-morbid conditions or underlying diseases. Peripheral manifestations and end-organ dysfunction are responsible for progression of symptoms that is inevitable despite optimal therapy. When symptoms are no longer controlled and patients become home bound, referral to a palliative care program will help patients deal with a hopeless situation.

In addition, there are changes in vascular endothelium, the layer of cells lining the inside of blood vessels, in heart failure. This leads to vasoconstriction, reduced blood flow and increased blood pressure. Endothelial cells in the heart also modulate myocardial function through direct interaction with cardiac myocytes. Such impairments in the endothelium are responsible for many of the manifestations of heart failure independent of cardiac pumping ability and must be addressed in therapy.

4.4. Life Expectancy

When compared to that of age and gender matched healthy subjects, the life expectancy of patients with CHF due to LV diastolic dysfunction is reduced although less markedly than that of patients with CHF due to LV systolic dysfunction (Kaminsky et al., 2000; Zile and Baicu, 2004). In general, systolic heart failure is associated with a 10 percent annual mortality; diastolic heart failure is associated with a lower annual mortality, which ranges from one-half to two-thirds of that of systolic heart failure. Evaluation of the effects of therapy on LV remodeling and functional capacity is critically important in considering referral to a palliative care program in patients with CHF. Lack of improvement in LV systolic function after long-term beta-adrenergic-blockade therapy or in functional capacity after long-term ACE inhibition suggests irreversibility and thereby a high likelihood of a progressive downhill course. Thus, referral to a palliative care program is appropriate when patients with severe CHF fail to improve or worsen while receiving optimal medical therapy. Three clinical conditions provide an ominous sign of markedly reduced life expectancy. First, patients with increasingly frequent hospitalizations despite strict adherence to a low-sodium diet and medications have a dismal prognosis. Second, failure to tolerate previously tolerated ACE inhibition or beta-adrenergic-blockade therapy usually indicates a life expectancy of less than 6-12 months. Third, non specific abdominal discomfort, in addition to common complaints of fatigue and dyspnea and a rising creatinine level (evidence of kidney dysfunction), serve as hints at intermittent bowel ischemia that in turn points to a low-output state. A low-output state despite optimal medical therapy clearly indicates a dismal prognosis as demonstrated in the conventional treatment arm of the Randomized Evaluation of Mechanical Assistance for the Treatment of Congestive Heart failure (REMATCH) trial. In the REMATCH trial, patients with end-stage CHF who were ineligible for transplantation were randomly assigned to receive an implantable left ventricular assist device or to optimal medical management Those with LVADs experienced significant improvement in one- or two-year survival, as well as improved quality of life, relative to optimal medical management (Rose et al., 2001).

The shorter is life expectancy, the greater is the emphasis on quality of life since interventions aimed at prolonging life are no longer relevant. A palliative care program designed for the last months of life may greatly help patients deal with a hopeless situation. Many patients remain in functional class III (NYHA) with periodic decline to functional class IV despite more intense care and especially relative to fluid control. Such patients may demonstrate a persistently reduced cardiac index and the ability to redistribute blood flow to essential organs as needed (heart, kidneys and brain) at the expense of other vascular beds especially cutaneous vascular beds. When this capacity for exquisite blood flow redistribution is lost, kidney function deteriorates, bowel ischemia develops and patients become bed-ridden. What triggers this catastrophic vascular event is unclear but clinically this resembles endotoxic shock. Palliative care at this point is inevitable and urgent.

In summary, progression of CHF due to LV systolic or diastolic dysfunction evolves in two stages. In response to acute injury or chronic overload the LV chamber undergoes hypertrophy and dilatation in order to maintain cardiac output in an attempt to return LV wall tension towards normal. When the LV remodeling process is exhausted, cardiac reserve is progressively lost with a reduced forward output at rest. Skeletal muscle alterations develop, systemic inflammation occurs and an impaired capacity to excrete sodium and toxic metabolites ensues. These peripheral manifestations of heart failure progress despite treatment and contribute to aggravate symptoms that were initially entirely related to LV dysfunction. The lack of reversibility of LV remodeling and peripheral manifestations and the failure to tolerate therapeutic interventions previously shown to be beneficial are unequivocal predictors of a poor outcome and the need to initiate a palliative care program.

5. Modes of Demise

In patients with CHF due to LV systolic dysfunction death can be sudden, due to a fatal cardiac arrhythmia, or progressive due to gradual decline in cardiac output and sodium and fluid excretory capacity. Sudden death is the mode of demise in 50% of patients with CHF resulting from LV systolic dysfunction (Lee et al., 2003). Sudden death is most often due to arrhythmias such as rapid ventricular tachycardia or fibrillation and occasionally to bradycardia or electro-mechanical dissociation. However, fatal arrhythmias may not be an isolated event but occur in the context of symptomatic progressive CHF. The success with an implantable cardiac defibrillator (ICD) for the treatment of ventricular tachycardia and ventricular fibrillation in patients with LV systolic dysfunction due to cardiomyopathy is presently shifting the mode of demise to progressive heart failure, since patients with systolic heart failure and ICD's are now protected from sudden death. However, ventricular arrhythmias in patients with end-stage systolic heart failure may be viewed as a blessing in disguise as ventricular arrhythmias protect patients who have an extremely limited life expectancy from a painful and slow death. In that regard, disabling the defibrillator function of an ICD may be part of a palliative care program aimed at improving the well being of patients with end stage systolic heart failure in the last days or weeks of life. Moreover the advantages and disadvantages of an ICD in a patient with CHF and symptoms compatible with NYHA functional class IV may best be discussed in the multidisciplinary framework of a palliative care program with the patient or his/her health care proxy. The therapeutic challenge when managing patients with CHF due to LV systolic function is to provide them with an acceptable level of functional status until the last few days of life while avoiding interventions that prolong life at the expense of physical discomfort or functional status. These are the same concerns faced by physicians caring for patients with other advanced illnesses such as terminal malignancy.

Sudden death is less likely in patients with diastolic heart failure than in patients with systolic heart failure. Thus steady progression of heart failure and flare ups of co-morbid conditions especially cerebrovascular accidents are mostly responsible for the demise of patients with diastolic heart failure. The presence of co-morbid conditions such as cerebrovascular disease, chronic obstructive lung disease, hepatic cirrhosis and dementia was shown to significantly contribute to the fatal outcome of patients with CHF hospitalized for heart failure (Fox *et al.*, 1999).

6. Timing of the Referral to a Palliative Care Program

6.1. Patients Managed Outside of a Heart Failure Program

The great majority of patients with CHF related to LV systolic dysfunction are managed by primary care physicians, internists or general cardiologists. This is especially the case for elderly patients with CHF due to LV diastolic dysfunction who are not evaluated for cardiac transplantation nor candidates for an implantable LV assist device according to the REMATCH trial criteria (Rose *et al.*, 2001). Although not routinely applied, algorithms for predicting prognosis are extremely useful in these circumstances to attract the attention of the caretaker to the limited life expectancy of his/her patient. An algorithm was derived from the National Hospice Organization guidelines and the Epidemiologie de l'Insuffisance Cardiaque Avancee en Lorraine (EPICAL) study by Albert and colleagues (Albert, 2002). The aim of the algorithm is to help physicians determine the most opportune time for referring patients with severe CHF to a palliative care program (Alla *et al.*, 2000). Albert and colleagues recommend a different algorithm in patients with ischemic and non-ischemic cardiomyopathy. Since differences in clinical profile and treatment that initially exist in patients with ischemic and non ischemic cardiomyopathy become blurred as these conditions progress one may question the need to use a different algorithm to determine the timing of a palliative care referral in patients with ischemic and non-ischemic cardiomyopathy. The following is adapted from the algorithm proposed by Albert and colleagues. It applies to patients with ischemic and non-ischemic cardiomyopathy. Only two of the four confirmatory criteria are required. The limited use of prognostic indices is notorious in clinical practice (Albert, 2002). Thus rather than recommending calculation of a prognostic score with numerical values that cannot be readily calculated by busy practitioners, the above mentioned criteria underline functional intolerance and end organ impairment. Referral to palliative care program should be considered when symptoms of patients with CHF clearly interfere in an unacceptable manner with their daily living despite adherence to heart failure guidelines and patients exhibit evidence of end organ dysfunction.

6.2. Patients Managed in a Heart Failure Program

The appropriate timing of a referral to a palliative care program is more flexible when patients with advanced CHF are managed in the framework of a specialized Heart Failure Program. The skills provided by the Heart Failure Program in controlling symptoms and the skills of the Palliative Care team in dealing with end-of-life decisions and coordinating home care services are complementary to provide an optimal quality of care to patients with limited life expectancy. Intensive homecare surveillance programs have been shown to reduce morbidity, rehospitalization and improve quality-of-life for patients with advanced CHF, this may represent good alternatives for patients who do not wish to be referred to hospice services or in whom life expectancy is estimated at more than six months. Such programs provide intensive patient and family education about the disease and symptom management, frequent nursing visits, check in phone calls on weekends, 24 hour, 7 day a week on-call service and access to an urgent medication kit in the home.The case management strategy, operating within a specialized heart failure program, include physician and patient education, promotion of intensive medical therapy and life-style modification, close patient monitoring, helping patients to cope with medical, insurance and emotional issues. Most case management programs for patients with heart failure are led by cardiologists and conducted by nurses and nurse practitioners. Studies demonstrated cost-effectiveness, and heart failure patients cared for by these programs had fewer hospital admissions. (Kornowski *et al.*, 1995; Pantilat and Steimle, 2004; Rich, 1999). With the increasing willingness of hospices in the era of *Open Access* to consider coverage of some high cost palliative care interventions: for example, biventricular cardiac pacing is effective in resynchronizing cardiac contraction. There is evidence that such interventions improve ventricular performance. For CHF patients the benefits include better exercise tolerance and better quality of life, and potentially lowering the NYHA severity classification. As a consequence increasing numbers of patients may be willing to consider enrollment in a hospice program (Saxon *et al.*, 1999; Gras *et al.*, 1998; Cohen and Klein, 2002).

As already mentioned, failure to tolerate previously tolerated therapy, back-to-back hospitalization despite full adherence to medications and diet, and the development of symptoms compatible with a low-flow state such as lethargy, non-specific abdominal pain and weight loss should prompt referral to a palliative care program. Similarly, steady deterioration of kidney function especially when not reversible by intravenous vasoactive or positive inotropic therapy should also prompt referral to a palliative care program. The criteria for timing the referral of patients managed in a heart failure program to a palliative care program are summarized in Table 8.1. Calculation of various algorithms aimed at predicting survival is most useful to confirm the clinical evaluation when patients are closely monitored in the framework of a heart failure program. Overall, algorithms provide a global snapshot assessment of the patient's clinical course while close follow up by experienced physicians or nurse practitioners allows detection of functional changes that point to limited life expectancy and the appropriateness of a referral to a palliative care program. When a patient is accepted by a palliative care program, he/she should continue to follow up with the heart failure program for continuity of care and prevention of a feeling of abandonment. Optimally, the care of patients conjointly managed by a heart failure and palliative care program should be discussed at monthly combined meetings. The relative emphasis on heart failure therapy versus comfort care can be then tailored according to his/her clinical course. A large heart failure program that cares for several hundred patients may include a palliative care specialist in their staff to help deal with end of life decisions and management that often overburden social workers.

TABLE 8.1. When to refer for palliative care program

Initial Criteria:
Functional status compatible with NYHA functional class IV
Functional deterioration despite optimal therapy as defined by current guidelines
All medical and surgical options have been exhausted or declined.
Home inotropic or vasoactive intravenous therapy required.
Inability to care for one's self due to lethargy, confusion, and intolerance to minimal physical activity or skeletal muscle wasting.

Confirmatory Criteria:
Hyponatremia <134 mmol/l
Tachycardia >110 beats/minute
Serum creatinine >2.5 mg/dL, evidence of kidney dysfunction.

Anemia: Hemoglobin <10 g/dL not responding to erythropoietin therapy to stimulate production of red blood cells.

6.3. Patients with Left Ventricular Assist Devices

Left Ventricular Assist Devices (LVAD's) are now a means to prolong life in patients with end-stage CHF who are not candidate for cardiac transplantation. This new indication for LVAD's is commonly referred to as "destination" therapy.The LVAD is a battery-operated mechanical pump-like device that is surgically implanted. It helps a weakened heart to maintain pumping ability. The only device currently approved by the FDA for destination therapy is the Heartmate. It has portable batteries and a controller that allows good mobility. The device prolongs life in patients with end stage CHF until sepsis or mechanical failure 20 to 24 months after implantation (Devereaux *et al.*, 2004; Rose *et al.*, 2001). Patients experienced on average two hospitalizations for sepsis requiring antibiotic therapy within 6 months of LVAD implantation. Anticoagulation is not required after Heartmate implantation. The rate of neurological events is four to five times more frequent with destination therapy than with optimal medical therapy but about eighty per cent of patients do not experience serious neurological events.

Thus implantation of a Heartmate clearly prolongs survival when compared to optimal therapy, despite a high rate of complications. Such a high rate of complications coupled to daily care of batteries and drive line is physically and psychologically draining for the patient and his/her spouse. In view of the demands that destination therapy may make on the patient and his/her family and the risk of an abrupt fatal event at any time, involvement with a palliative care program appears judicious once the acute period post surgical period is over. From a legal standpoint, life-sustaining device cannot be turned off without clear knowledge and documentation of the patient desire to discontinue mechanical support in pre-specified situations. Discussion with the patient about circumstances that could lead to discontinuation of support can be made easier by involvement of a third party such as a palliative care team. Destination therapy is in its nature essentially palliative. The duration of the device is finite and the patient is well aware of it. End-of-life decisions can be made by following well-established bioethical principles when working closely with a palliative care program. Destination therapy commonly entails difficult decisions that require close collaboration between heart failure and palliative care specialists. Involvement of a palliative care team at early stage after implantation of the device even in the absence of complications is an efficient and humane way to deal with a situation that sooner or later will exhaust the most dedicated cardiologists and cardiothoracic surgeons. In a larger sense the considerations for palliative care for patients with end-stage CHF are essentially the same as those for patients with end-stage malignancy. When life can no longer be sustained in acceptable manner, the comfort and ease of patients becomes the primary concern. Smaller and more efficient auxiliary pumps provided partial cardiac output support are being developed. This will make destination therapy more common and the end-points for palliative care a more urgent issue.

7. Summary

End-stage heart failure implies a very limited life expectancy and thereby involves end-of-life decisions that are better handled in collaboration with a palliative care program. Thus the real issue is not whether patients with CHF should be referred to a palliative care program but when they should be referred. Discerning that patients with CHF are in the last weeks to months of their life is made difficult by the symptomatic peaks and troughs that characterize the evolution of CHF. Nevertheless, physical deterioration leading to incapacity of performing basic daily activities without help is a definite indication for referral to a palliative care program in patients with CHF.

Glossary

Left Ventricular Assist Device: implanted mechanical devices which include a prosthetic left ventricle. Devices include the Heartmate I and II, Novacor, Thoratec, Abiomed pumps. The major indication is cardiogenic shock that is refractory to inotropes and intraaortic balloon pumping. They are usually used as a bridge to cardiac transplantation or may be implanted as permanent devices "destination therapy".

Myocardium: The cardiac muscle.

Systole: Contraction of the cardiac muscle.

Diastole: Relaxation of the cardiac muscle.

Unloading agents: Medications which reduce peripheral arterial resistance to cardiac contraction and pumping action. An example would be enalapril which is an angiotensin converting enzyme inhibitor medication (ACE inhibitor).

Peak Aerobic Capacity: Maximum oxygen consumption.

Myocardial infarction: Colloquially known as a heart attack. Loss of coronary arterial blood supply to a region of the heart muscle (cardiac ischemia) which is accompanied by death of heart muscle cells. It is typically associated with chest pain and can be associated with cardiogenic shock and cardiac arrhythmias.

Left Ventricular hypertrophy: Thickening of the muscle of the left ventricle.

Ventricular Remodeling: Alteration in the size, shape and function of the ventricle which may ultimately result in reduced contractility.

Myocardial fibrosis: Scarring of the heart muscle.

Endotoxic Shock: Seen in gram negative bacterial sepsis. It is characterized by fever, muscle breakdown, prolonged clotting and low blood pressure.

Cardiac arrhythmias: Abnormalities of the cardiac rhythm that can result in cardiovascular arrest or cardiac arrest. They include ventricular tachycardia (a rapid and regular ventricular rhythm), ventricular fibrillation (a rapid and irregular ventricular rhythm) bradycardia (an abnormally slow cardiac rhythm) and electromechanical disassociation (absence of cardiac mechanical activity in the presence of a cardiac rhythm).

Implantable Cardiac Defibrillator: implantable devices that promptly detect and correct ventricular arrhythmias. They are indicated for ventricular tachycardia that is accompanied by hemodynamic instability or ventricular fibrillation that doesn't respond to medications.

Vasoactive agent: An agent that's mechanism of action is mediated in the blood vessels.

Positive inotrope: an agent which enhances cardiac contractility and pumping ability.

Beta Adrenergic blockade: Use of drugs which antagonize the cardiovascular effects of catecholamines in hypertension, angina pectoris and cardiac arrhythmia. They can decrease the heart rate, blood pressure and myocardial contractility. Such medications include propranolol and metoprolol.

Cardiac Cachexia: Occurs in severe heart failure and is characterized by serious weight loss because of elevation of tumor necrosis factor and increased metabolic rate. It is also associated with nausea, loss of appetite due to congestion of the liver and the effects of medications and abdominal fullness as well as decreased intestinal absorption due to congestion in the intestinal veins.

Hyponatremia is an abnormally low concentration of sodium in the blood. This may occur in kidney, liver or heart failure or with excessive hydration. The normal serum (blood) concentration of sodium is 135 to 145 mEq/l.

Creatinine is a breakdown product of creatine, which is an important part of muscle. A serum creatinine test measures the amount of creatinine in the blood. The test is performed to evaluate kidney function. If kidney function is abnormal, creatinine levels will increase in the blood, due to decreased excretion (removal from the body) of creatinine in the urine. A normal (usual) value is 0.8 to 1.4 mg/dl.

Anemia is a common blood disorder in which there are not enough red blood cells to carry oxygen to the tissues. It is measured with a red blood cell count or hemoglobin level. *Hemoglobin* is the protein that carries oxygen in the blood. It is contained in red blood cells. Both high and low hemoglobin counts indicate defects in the balance of red blood cells in the blood, and may indicate disease. The normal red blood cell count for a male is : 4.7 to 6.1 million cells/mcl and for a female: 4.2 to 5.4 million cells/mcl Normal levels of hemoglobin in a male are 13.8 to 17.2 g/dl and 12.1 to 15.1g/dl in females.

Erythropoietin is a hormone that is produced by oxygen sensitive cells in the kidney in response to reductions in the oxygen content of the blood. Synthetic forms of this hormone are used to treat anemia in chronic diseases including chronic renal failure, cancer and congestive heart failure.

Cardiomyopathy any weakening or loss of function of the heart muscle with resultant loss of cardiac pumping of blood through the lungs and the rest of the body.

Renin Angiotensin System Renin is an enzyme that is released by cells of the juxtaglomerular apparatus of the kidney into the blood in response to low sodium or low blood volume. Renin promotes the conversion of Angiotensinogen (a protein released into the blood by the liver to Angiotensin I). Angiotensin I is converted to Angiotensin II by enzymes, which are located in the veins of the lungs. Angiotensin II acts on the cortex of the adrenal glands to promote the release of Aldosterone. Aldosterone acts within the kidneys to decrease the loss of sodium ions and fluid. Angiotensin also causes blood vessels to constrict (narrow). This results in increased blood pressure. Angiotensin II is a growth factor that can lead to eventual cardiac deterioration. Activation of this system represents an adverse prognostic marker in CHF. The Angiotensin Converting Enzyme Inhibitor medications (captopril and lisinopril) decrease the levels of serum Angiotensin II and Aldosterone and promote vasodilation (increase in the size of the

blood vessels), which lowers the blood pressure and reduces the workload of the heart and the Angiotensin Receptor Blockers (losartan, valsartan, irbesartan and candasartan) are commonly used in the treatment of CHF. The Angiotensin Receptor Blockers prevent Angiotensin II from binding with the Angiotensin II receptor in blood vessels and the heart. This stops the blood pressure from rising.

Vasodilators include isosorbide dinitrate, nesiritide, hydralazine, angiotensin converting enzyme inhibitors, nitrates and minoxidil. They cause the blood vessel wall to relax. This allows blood to flow more easily and can result in reductions in blood pressure.

Endothelium is the smooth inner lining of many structures including the blood vessels and heart (endomyocardium). CHF patients have impaired endothelial-dependent vasodilation. It is thought to relate to decreased endothelial derived production of nitric oxide in the blood vessels and the heart. Endothelial function in CHF patients can be improved with certain medications including the Angiotensin Converting Enzyme Inhibitor medications. There is some evidence to suggest that the lipid lowering statin medications (hydorxy 3 methyl glutaryl coenzyme A reductase inhibitor medications) can also beneficially modulate nitric oxide levels and reduce platelet activation in experimental CHF models.

References

2001 Heart and Stroke Statistical Update Dallas: American Heart Association, 2000, permanent.access.gpo.gov/lps6793/www.americanheart.org/catalog/scientific_catpage70.html

Alla, F., Briancon, S., Julliere, Y., Mertes, P.M., Villemot, J.P., and Zannad, F. (2000). Differential Clinical Prognostic Classification in Dilated and Ischemic Advanced Heart Failure. *American Heart Journal.* 139:895-904.

American Heart Association: 1998 Heart and stroke statistical update. American Heart Association, Dallas, Tx 1998, www.mplsheartfoundation.org/news/annualreport/ar_1998.asp

American Heart Association/ American College of Cardiology Guidelines Update 2005. The diagnosis and management of chronic heart failure in the adult, americanheart.org/presenter.jhtml?identifier=3036136.

Cohen, T.J. and Klein, J. (2002). Cardiac resynchronization therapy for treatment of chronic heart failure. *Journal of Invasive Cardiology.* 14(1):48-53.

Devereux, R.B., Watchell, K., Gerdts, E., Boman, K., Nieminen, M.S., Papademetriou, V., Rokkedal, J., Harris, K., Aurup, P., and Dahlof, B. (2004). Prognostic significance of left ventricular mass change during treatment of hypertension. *Journal of the American Medical Association.* 292:2350-2356.

Fox, E., Landrun-McNiff, K., Zhong, Z., Dawson, N.V., Wu, A.W., Lynn, J., for the SUPPORT Investigators. (1999). Evaluation of prognostic criteria for determining hospice eligibility in patients with advanced lung, heart, or liver disease. *Journal of the American Medical Association.* 282:1638-1645.

Hanratty, B., Hibbert, D., Mair, F., May, C., Ward, C., Capewell, S., Litva, A., and Corcoran, G. (2002). Doctors' perceptions of palliative care for heart failure: focus group study. *British Medical Journal.* 325(7364):581-5.

Garg, R., Packer, M., Pitt, B., and Yusuf, S. (1993). Heart failure in the 1990's:evaluation of a major public health problem in cardiovascular medicine. *Journal of the American College of Cardiology.* 22:3-5A (Suppl A).

Gras, D., Mabo, P., Tang, T., and Skehan, D. (1998). Multisite pacing as a supplemental treatment of congestive heart failure: preliminary results of the medtronic inc. insync study. *Pacing and Clinical Electrophysiology.* 21(11Pt2):2249-55.

Graves, E.J. (1992). Detailed diagnoses and procedures. National Hospital Discharge Survey, 1990 Vital and health statistics, series 13, data from the National Health Survey. National Center for Health Statistics, Hyattsville, MD,; pp. 113:1-225.

Jiang, W., Alexander, J., and O'Connor, M. (2001). Relationship of depression to increased risk of mortality and rehospitalization in patients with congestive heart failure. *Archives of Internal Medicine.* 161:1849-1856.

Kaminsky, L.A., Brubaker, P.H., Peaker, B., and Kitzman, D.W. (2000). Prediction of peak oxygen uptake from cycle exercise test work level in heart failure patients 65 years of age. *The American Journal of Cardiology.* 85:1385-1387.

Kitzman, D.W., Little, W.C., Brubaker, P.H., and Stewart, K.P. (2002). Pathophysiological characterization of isolated diastolic heart failure in comparison to isolated systolic heart failure. *Journal of the American Medical Association.* 288:2144-2150.

Koenig, H.G. (1998). Depression in hospitalized older patients with congestive heart failure. *General Hospital Psychiatry.* 20:29-43.

Kornowski, R., Zeeli, D., Averbuch, M., Pines, A., Finkelstein, A., Schwartz, D.Moshkovitz, M., Weinreb, B., and Miller M (1995). Intensive home-care and surveillance prevents hospitalization and improves morbidity rates among elderly patients with severe congestive heart failure. *American Heart Journal.* 129(4):762-6.

Lee, D.S., Austin, P.C., Rouleau, J.L., Liu, P.P., Naimark, D., and Tu, J.V. (2003). Predicting mortality among patients hospitalized for heart failure. *Journal of the American Medical Association.* 290:2581-2587.

Levenson, J.W., McCarthy, E.P., Lynn, J., Davis, R.B., and Phillips, R.S. (2000). The last six months of life for patients with congestive heart failure. *Journal of the American Geriatric Society.* 48(Suppl 5):S101-S109.

Lynn, J., Teno, J.M., and Phillips, R.S. (1997). Perceptions of the family members of the dying experiences older seriously ill patients. *Annals of Internal Medicine.* 126(2):97-106.

McAlister, F.A., Teo, K.K., and Taher, M. (1999). Insights into the contemporary epidemiology and outpatient management of congestive heart failure. *American Heart Journal.* 138(1pt1):87-94.

McCarthy, M., Lay, M., and Addington-Hall, J. (1996). Dying from heart disease. *Journal of the Royal College of Physicians in London.* 30:325-328.

Murray, S.A., Boyd, K., Kendall, M., Worth, A., Benton, T.F., and Clausen, H. (2002). Dying of lung cancer or cardiac failure: prospective qualitative interview study of patients and their caregivers in the community. *British Medical Journal.* 325(7370):929.

O'Connell, J.B. and Bristow, M.R. (1994). Economic impact of heart failure in the United States: time for a different approach. *Journal of Heart and Lung Transplant.* 13:S107-12.

Pantilat, S.Z., and Steimle, A.E. (2004). Palliative care for patients with heart failure; *Journal of the American Medical Association.* 291:2476-2482.

Pyenson, B., Connor, S., Fitch, K. and Kinzbrunner, B. (2004). Medicare costs in matched hospice and non-hospice cohorts. *Journal of Pain and Symptom Management.* 28(3):200-210.

Rich, M.W., Heart failure disease management: a critical review. (1999). *Journal of Cardiac Failure.* 5(1):64-75.

Rose, E.A., Gelijns, A.C., and Moskowitz, A.J. (2001). Long-term mechanical left ventricular assistance for end-stage heart failure. *New England Journal of Medicine.* 345:1435-1443.

Saxon, L.A., Boehmer, J.P., and Daoud, E. (1999). Biventricular pacing in patients with congestive heart failure : two prospective randomized trials. The VIGOR CHF and *VENTAK CHF investigators. American Journal of Cardiology.* 11:83 (5B): 120D-123D.

The SOLVD investigators. (1992). Effect of enalapril on mortality and the development of heart failure in asymptomatic patients with reduced left ventricular ejection fraction. *New England Journal of Medicine.* 327:685-691.

Stevenson, W.G., Stevenson, L.W. (2001). Prevention of sudden death in heart failure. *Journal of Cardiovascular Electrophysiology.* 1:112-114.

SUPPORT Principal Investigators. (1995). A controlled trial to improve care for seriously ill hospitalized patients. *Journal of the American Medical Association.* 274:1591-1598.

Zile, M.R. and Baicu, C.F. (2004). Alterations in ventricular function: diastolic heart failure Mann DL (ed.), *Heart failure: a companion to Braunwald's Heart Disease, Saunders, Publishing, Philadelphia, PA.* pp. 209-227.

9
Palliative Care for Patients with Alzheimer's Dementia: Advance Care Planning Across Transition Points

Jennifer Rhodes-Kropf MD

Alzheimer's Dementia (AD) is the most prevalent progressive neurodegenerative disease. It begins with minute memory impairment and ultimately leads to the loss of all mental and physical function. A person with AD lives an average of eight years from diagnosis and could live as many as 20 years (Odle, 2003). By the year 2000, there were about 4.5 million in the U.S. population with A.D, with one in 10 persons over the age of 65, and nearly half of those over 85 having AD By 2050, the number is projected to increase to 13.2 million (Hebert *et al.*, 2003). Since there is no cure for AD, "persons with AD need interventions that are directed to relief of suffering, pain control, and comfort, often associated with 'palliative' rather than . . . curative measures.' This chapter is intended to assist health care administrators, health care planners, and public policy professionals to make policy decisions that may improve quality of life for those afflicted with AD and that may minimize the burden of care on family and loved ones. The authors trace the illness through transition points and discuss advance care planning and palliative care- focusing on issues specific to patients with AD.

The natural history or progression of disease depends on the dementia type. The distinguishing characteristics of AD are the presence of two abnormalities in the brain; amyloid plaques and neurofibriallry tangles. Amyloid plaques, in the tissue between nerve cells. Are composed of the protein beta-amyloid with degenerating parts of neurons and other cells. Researchers do not know if amyloid plaques or neurofibrillary tangles are harmful, or consequences of the disease process that damages neurons and leads to symptoms of AD. A study by Marshall *et al.* (2006) revealed a correlation between decline in activities of daily living or ADL scores and higher plaque and neurofibrillary tangle counts suggesting a "greater overall pathologic burden".

JENNIFER RHODES-KROPF • Montefiore Medical Center, 111th East 210th Street, Bronx, New York 10467

About 60 to 80% of dementia patients have AD (Shadlen and Larson, 2004). Vascular dementia is the second most common cause of dementia, accounting for up to 20% of all dementias. Vascular dementia is caused by brain damage from cerebrovascular or cardiovascular disease. While AD progresses gradually over time, symptoms of vascular dementia often begin suddenly, frequently after a stroke, and typically progresses in a step-wise manner. This means that there is a decline in memory and function, which remains at a stable level until the next vascular insult when the next plateau in memory and function is reached. By contrast AD progresses gradually over time.

Other forms of dementia include Lewy body dementia (about 10%), dementia due to Parkinson's disease (about 5%), and the small remainder of patients have dementia resulting from alcohol abuse, medication side effects, depression and other central nervous system illnesses (Shadlen and Larosn, 2004; Rahkonen *et al.*, 2003).

Nevertheless, the ultimate deficits and co-morbidities of these dementing illnesses are the same and typically include paucity of speech, aphasia (difficulty speaking), an inability to recognize family members, impaired ambulation, urinary and fecal incontinence, anorexia, dysphasia (difficulty swallowing), weight loss, pressure sores, and pneumonia. Pneumonia is the most frequent immediate cause of death in AD (Molsa *et al.*, 1986; Volicer *et al.*, 2001).

Mild cognitive impairment is defined as cognitive decline greater than expected for an individual's age but that does not interfere notably with activities of daily life. While some individuals with mild cognitive impairment appear to remain stable over time, it is relevant that possibly more than half may progress to dementia within five years. The International Psychogeriatric Association Expert Conference to review available data on mild cognitive impairment was convened in Bethesda, Maryland, January 2005. According to the proceedings mild cognitive impairment portends a high risk of progression. Mild cognitive impairment may represent a prodromal stage of AD, and its identification could facilitate secondary prevention.

Although, this chapter focuses specifically on the issues that arise as AD progresses, the same management principles may be applied to patients with other types of dementia.

AD is a clinical diagnosis that is based upon criteria defined by the Diagnostic and Statistical Manual of Mental Disorders, 4th ed. (American Psychiatric Association, 1994). These criteria include impairments in short and long term memory that are severe enough to interfere with work or usual social activities.

Diagnosis is made by a physician experienced in the assessment of dementia who obtains information from a close family member or friend regarding the patient's ability to function. Mental status tests are also administered. These clinical assessment methods are time consuming, yet can provide predictive accuracy rates of 85% to 90% for AD (Morris, 2003).

The gradual decline in health for patients with AD varies from individual to individual, but typically the first evidence of decline is marked by impairment in executive function or the instrumental activities of daily living (IADLs) such as bill paying, shopping, and cooking. The individual may get lost while driving or taking the bus. Additionally, there may be new depression, changes in personality, and behavioral problems such as paranoia or agitation.

The individual may or may not be aware of his/her new deficits or psychiatric problems. Often family brings the person to the doctor for an evaluation because they notice some of these initial problems. It is important, in the early stage of AD, to educate family about the natural history of AD so that they know what to expect, and to permit planning for the future. This planning should include designation of a health care proxy, completion of a living will, and designation of a durable power of attorney to manage finances. It is also advised, that the patient and family meet with an elder lawyer or estate planner to try and protect spousal assets. Furthermore, it is helpful to the patient, family and medical science, to discuss with the patient early on in the disease, whether or not the patient wishes to donate his or her brain upon death to further medical research.

There is no cure for AD. However, data show that some agents (cholinesterase inhibitors) may slow AD progression, but provide at best only minimal improvement in memory (Cummings, 2004). Data also suggest that cholinesterase inhibitors may enable AD patients to have fewer behavioral changes, maintain their ability to care for themselves, be less burdensome to caregivers, and defer their placement in nursing homes (Cummings, 2004). Of note, these drugs are costly, particularly to patients whose insurance does not cover medications.

Aside from medication, even though evidence is limited in terms of impact on AD progression, individuals should be encouraged to continue to be both physically and mentally active. As for vascular dementia, it now appears that some forms of vascular dementia may be preventable with the control of vascular risk factors, in particular hypertension, high cholesterol levels, and diabetes.

There comes a point in the illness when the individual's functional losses make safety a particular concern. For instance, it may no longer be safe for her to drive because she gets lost and has poor judgment. Also, there may be concern that she no longer can live at home because she may leave the stove burner or iron on, or if there were a fire that she would not be able to get out of the building independently. Home assistance or an assisted living residence may be needed, and ultimately 24 hour home care or nursing home placement.

Unfortunately, Medicare insurance does not pay for home services for patients who need help with personal care needs, unless the patients predicted survival is less than six months and thus she would qualify for the Medicare hospice benefit. Of note, patients who are poor enough to qualify for Medicaid insurance can get a home health aide for help with personal care. Otherwise people must pay for this custodial care "out of pocket."

Families should be referred to their local Department for the Aging program social workers as well as social workers at the Alzheimer's Foundation who can direct families to services in their areas based on their needs. These services include Meals on Wheels, Senior Center Programs, and Day Programs for the elderly. Please refer to the chapter on case management and the elderly.

A major issue of concern for families and health care providers is the management of psychiatric problems associated with AD. These include delusions, hallucinations, depression, anxiety and agitation (Head, 2003).

Environmental, behavioral, and communication modification should always be the first recourse for paranoid, agitated or anxious patients. Families and/or staff caring for patients with these issues benefit from specialized training. But measures based on these strategies may not be sufficient to protect patients who are a danger to themselves or others. If this is the case then the use of medication is recommended.

Depression is very prevalent among patients with AD. This is particularly true early in the illness, but it may develop at any time. Antidepressant medications are warranted (Head, 2003).

The final stages of AD are marked by functional losses in self-care or Activities of Daily Living (ADLs). These include toileting, dressing, bathing, and self-feeding. These losses also frequently occur concurrently with a paucity of speech, aphasia (difficulty in speaking), an inability to recognize family members, impaired ambulation, urinary and fecal incontinence, anorexia, dysphasia (difficulty swallowing), weight loss, recurrent pneumonia, and often pressure sores (decubiti). As has been mentioned earlier, these symptoms are also common in other forms of dementia.

The functional status and behavior of the patient are major determinants of nursing home placement. As demonstrated by researchers Heyman et al. (1997) and Porsteinsson et al. (2001), patient variables include severity of cognitive impairment, inability to perform self-care tasks, incontinence, sleep/wake cycle disturbances, and behavioral changes.

With the progressive development of multiple impairments in AD patients, caring for a relative with AD takes a huge toll on the caregiver physically, emotionally, and financially. Thus, the capabilities and time commitments of caregivers also play an important role in whether or not individuals with dementia are placed in a nursing home and at what point in the disease placement occurs. Cohen et al. (1993) prospectively studied the factors determining the decision to institutionalize dementing individuals. Predictors of placement included younger caregivers, their need to work outside of the home, and caring for more than one person (Cohen et al., 1993). One randomized, controlled trial showed that a structured, continuous, caregiver support program can delay nursing home placement (Mittelman et al., 1996). A controlled study of respite services for caregivers of AD patients demonstrated that families with respite care maintained their relative significantly longer in the community (22 days) (Lawton et al., 1989).

The patient's physician should also discuss "goals of care" with his family before the disease is in its advanced stages; before the onset of losses in ADLs. The "goals of care" for the patient in the advanced stages of AD should focus on comfort. In other words, so as not to burden the patient, medical testing and interventions should only occur if it is likely that the testing and interventions will result in improved quality of life. This philosophy should also guide the management of all problems that arise.

Consistent with the goal of comfort is the recommendation that a DNR (Do Not Resuscitate) order be issued. Appelbaum *et al.* (1990) reviewed outcomes of attempted cardiopulmonary resuscitation by pre-hospital ambulance crews where CPR was initiated in a nursing home, compared to attempted CPR in non-residents. Only 2% (2/117) of nursing home patients and 11% (61/580) nonresidents survived until discharge from the hospital. Of the two nursing home patients who survived, one spent 30 days in the hospital and died 8 months after returning to the nursing home demented, cachetic and with a large sacral pressure sore. The other patient spent 60 days in the hospital and died 14 days after returning to the nursing home. The researchers concluded that "the benefits of cardiopulmonary resuscitation initiated in nursing homes are extremely limited" (Applebaum *et al.*, 1990).

One of the most challenging issues faced by the family and physician caring for a patient with advanced AD is that of anorexia and dysphasia. A commonly asked question asked, by families of physicians is "Are you going to let my mother starve to death?" This question has two aspects; 1) Does tube feeding the patient with AD prolong life via caloric support? 2) Does tube feeding the patient with AD enhance quality of life or reduce suffering? In regards to the former, non-randomized, retrospective studies have found no survival advantage for feeding tubes in patients with dementia (Finucane *et al.*, 1999). This may be contrasted with research that has found that the use of feeding tubes in patients with such reversible conditions as early stage head and neck cancer prolonged life.

It is important to note that most dying patients do *not* experience hunger or thirst. Although dry mouth is a common problem, it is usually multifactorial and not relieved by artificial hydration (Finucane *et al.*, 1999). Although the literature is limited to a few observational studies, there are no studies that demonstrate that the use of tube feeding improves the quality of life. It may make quality of life worse because of an increased need for physical restraints (some patients try to pull out the tube) pain, infections, "indignity" cost, and the denial of the pleasure of eating (Finucane *et al.*, 1999).

Another question related to tube feeding, in the setting of anorexia and dysphasia, is whether or not tube feeding is a means to prevent aspiration pneumonia. No study has demonstrated a reduction in the incidence of pneumonia through tube feeding. There are no published randomized control studies of this question. But we have had three retrospective studies comparing patients with and without tube feeding which showed that tube feeding did not reduce the incidence of pneumonia (Finucane and Bynum, 1996).

And there are many observational studies demonstrating a high rate of aspiration pneumonia in patients who are tube fed (Finucane *et al.*, 1999).

There are some measures that families and health care providers can take to try to decrease anorexia and improve calorie intake. A trial of megestorol acetate or the antidepressant medication mirtazapine may stimulate appetite (Morley, 2002). Families should also be encouraged to bring the person's favorite food to the nursing home or hospital. It is unfortunate that most nursing homes and hospitals do not serve "ethnic" foods. This problem of dietary preferences can contribute to low food intake. Other beneficial measures include ensuring that patients eat in a group setting, that staff spends enough time feeding those who need assistance, that there is a minimum of distraction that surroundings are pleasant, that family are present at meal times, that patients are fed as soon as they are seated, that their favorite music is played, and so forth. The provision of supplemental calorie drinks or puddings between meals is also recommended (Head, 2003).

The prediction of survival in end-stage dementia is challenging. In contrast to patients with terminal cancer, in which decline is typically a straight downward course, the disease trajectory for patients with end-stage dementia is marked by "ups and downs" (Lunney *et al.*, 2003). Researchers have, however, made some strides in prognostication in end-stage dementia. Early research by Volicer *et al.* (1993) demonstrated a relationship between severity of Alzheimer's dementia and development of fevers. Furthermore, their research revealed that older age at the time of occurence of fever, an antibiotic free management strategy, and nursing home admission within 6 months, were associated with a higher 6-month mortality (Volicer *et al.*, 1993). More recent research by Morrison and Siu (2000) compared the survival of cognitively intact to cognitively impaired individuals aged 70 and older who were hospitalized for pneumonia or hip fracture. End-stage dementia patients who received usual care in a hospital setting for either pneumonia or hip fracture had a four fold increase in 6-month mortality compared to their cognitively intact counterparts (Morrison and Siu, 2000).

The National Hospice and Palliative Care Organization (NHPCO) is particularly concerned with the development of accurate prediction tools for survival of dementia patients since patients need to be given a prognosis of six months or less to qualify for the Medicare Hospice Benefit. The NHPCO Guidelines for Determining Prognosis in Dementia combine functional assessment staging and the presence of medical co-morbidities (Stuart *et al.*, 1998) (Table 9.2). The functional assessment staging instrument (FAST) has the user rate the patient's level of disability in order of increasing severity from 1 to 7F (Table 9.1) (Reisberg, 1988). Currently, the NHPCO recommends stage 7A as an enrollment cut-off point for hospice care. In addition, the patient needs to have medical complications related to dementia and be non-ambulatory. Of note, researchers evaluated the mean survival time once stage 7C is reached, which was the NHPCO's previous cut off, Luchins *et al.* demonstrated a mean survival time of 6.9 months and

TABLE 9.1. Functional assessment staging (FAST): check highest consecutive level of disability

1. No difficulty either subjectively or objectively
2. Complaints that locations of objects have been forgotten, subjective work difficulties
3. Decreased job functioning evident to coworkers, difficulty in traveling to new locations, decreased organizational capacity*
4. Decreased ability to perform complex tasks (e.g., planning dinner for guests, handling personal finances such as forgetting to pay bills, difficulty marketing etc)
5. Required assistance in choosing proper clothing to wear for the day, season, or occasion (e.g., patients may wear the same clothing repeatedly unless supervised)*
6. A) Improperly putting on clothes without assistance or cuing (e.g., may put street clothes on over night clothes, put shoes on wrong feet, or have difficulty buttoning clothing) occasionally or more frequently over the past weeks*
   B) Unable to bathe properly (e.g., difficulty adjusting bath-water temperature) occasionally or more frequently over the past weeks*
   C) Inability to handle mechanics of toileting (e.g., forgets to flush toilet, does not wipe properly or properly dispose of toilet tissue) occasionally or more frequently over the past few weeks*
   D) Urinary incontinence (occasionally or more frequently over the past weeks)*
   E) Fecal incontinence (occasionally or more frequently over the past weeks)*
7. A) Ability to speak limited to approximately a half-dozen different intelligible words or fewer in the course of an average day or in the course of an intensive interview
   B) Speech ability limited to the use of a single intelligible word in an average day or in the course of an intensive interview (e.g., the person may repeat the word over and over)
   C) Loss of ambulatory ability (e.g., the individual cannot walk without personal assistance)
   D) Inability to sit up without assistance (e.g., the individual will fall over if there are not lateral rests [arms] on the chair)
   E) Loss of ability to smile
   F) Loss of ability to hold up head independently

* Scored primarily on the basis of information obtained from a knowledgeable informant and/or category.
Source: Reisberg

Hanrahan *et al.* demonstrated a mean survival time of 4.1 months (Luchins *et al.*, 1997; Hanrahan *et al.*, 1999).

However, these NHPCO guidelines for prognostication are too limited for many patients. Luchins *et al.* and Hanrahan *et al.* determined that about 50 to 60% of patients do not decline in the step by step manner described in FAST (Luchins *et al.*, 1997; Hanrahan *et al.*, 1999). Researchers need to continue to develop prognostication guidelines to assist health care providers in enrolling patients in hospice. And other obstacles to the enrollment of advanced dementia patients in hospice also need exploration, as until recently only 1% of patients in hospice care have a diagnosis of dementia (Hanrahan Luchins, 1995).

Should patients in their final stages of AD be admitted to the hospital and/or given antibiotics when there is an acute illness or infection? These are important issues that doctors should discuss with families as part of "goals of care." If it is decided that the "goals of care" should focus solely on comfort,

TABLE 9.2. National hospice and palliative care organization medical guidelines for determining prognosis in dementia

I. Functional Assessment Staging (FAST)
    A. May have a prognosis of up to 2 years. Survival time depends on variables such as the incidence of co-morbidities and the comprehensiveness of care.
    B. Is at or beyond stage 7 of the FAST scale.
    C. Displays *all* of the following characteristics:
        1. Unable to ambulate without assistance
        2. Unable to dress without assistance
        3. Unable to bathe properly
        4. Urinary and fecal incontinence
            a. Occasionally or more frequently, over the past weeks
            b. Reported by knowledgeable informant or caregiver
        5. Unable to speak or communicate meaningfully
            a. Ability to speak is limited to approximately a half dozen or fewer intelligible and different words, in the course of an average day or in the course of an intensive interview
II. Presence of medical complications
    A. Has displayed co morbid conditions of sufficient severity to warrant medical treatment, documented within the past year.
    B. Co morbid conditions associated with dementia:
        1. Aspiration pneumonia
        2. Pyelonephritis or upper urinary tract infection
        3. Septicemia
        4. Decubitus ulcers, multiple, stage 3-4
        5. Fever recurrent after antibiotics
    C. Difficulty swallowing food or refusal to eat, sufficiently severe that patient cannot maintain sufficient fluid and calorie intake to sustain life, with patient or surrogate refusing tube feeding or parenteral nutrition.
        1. Patients who are receiving tube feedings must have documented impaired nutritional status as indicated by:
            a. Unintentional, progressive weight loss of greater than 10% over the prior six months.
            b. Serum albumin less than 2.5 mg/dl may be a helpful prognostic indicator, but should not be used by itself.

Source: National Hospice and Palliative Care Organization.

then in the setting of most acute illnesses the person should be made comfortable at home or in the nursing home without admission to the hospital. This is because hospitalization for older patients, particularly those with cognitive impairment, can be hazardous. These hazards include delirium, pressure sores, functional decline, new incontinence, and nosocomial infections.

Once advanced dementia patients are admitted to the hospital they are often subjected to invasive and nonpalliative treatments (defined as treatments which were associated with risk and not provided to produce palliation) (Ahronheim et al., 1996). In this retrospective chart review of 164 patients (80 with dementia and 84 with cancer), 47% received invasive non-palliative treatments. There were no statistical differences in the use of non-palliative treatments between patients with dementia and patients with metastatic cancer. Patients with dementia were more likely to have complex noninvasive diagnostic tests. Eighty-eight percent received anotbiotics, often empirically, but patients with dementia were more likely to receive antibiotics for an identifiable infection. (Morrison *et al.*, 1998). If the goal is to achieve comfort at the end of life, the authors note, "then one should consider that serious infection may produce sedation and coma, allowing the patient a peaceful death, whereas antibiotics can awaken the terminally ill patient and prolong the process of dying."

A study of nursing home residents with pneumonia suggest that there may be less functional decline or death in the two months after the resolution of pneumonia in patients who are not transferred to the hospital (Fried *et al.*, 1997).

Lastly, it is important to discuss with the patient's family where they believe the patient would want to die. Unfortunately, most Americans die in an austere hospital environment.

Another issue for individuals with advanced dementia and a public health concern is the use of antibiotics for acute illness. Data suggest that survival is enhanced for patients with end-stage dementia receiving antibiotics for a febrile episode is limited (Hanrahan and Luchins, 1995; Muder *et al.*, 1996; Volicer, 1993; Fabiszewski *et al.*, 1990). Additionally, negative consequences for individuals receiving antibiotics can include: the pain of intravenous line placement, infection and blood clots at intravenous line sites, clostridium difficile infection (c. difficule causing diarrhea or colitis, allergic reactions, increased use of invasive tests, and increased use of mechanical restraints to prevent the patient from removing the intravenous line.

Lastly, the excessive use of antibiotics can increase the number of resistant bacterial infections and may prolong life for only a very short period of time, but at great expense (Diekema *et al.*, 2004).

Thus, the decision to hospitalize or give a patient antibiotics should not be automatic or capricous. It is often time consuming, but nonetheless there needs to be frequent and open dialogue with families about the patient's care plan.

The final palliative care element, and possibly the most important, for patients with dementia is the adequate management of pain. The prevalence of pain in several nursing home populations, in which the vast majority of patients are cognitively impaired, has been reported to be as high as 45% to 80% (Ferrell a,b, 1995). In the inpatient setting Morrison and Siu, 2000, compared pain and its treatment in advanced dementia and cognitively intact patients with hip fracture. Advanced dementia patients received one-third the amount of opioid analgesia as compared to cognitively intact subjects-40% of whom reported severe pain postoperatively. This suggested strongly that the majority of dementia patients were in severe pain postoperatively. Of note, only 24% of patients with end-stage dementia and hip fracture received a standing order for analgesics (Morrison and Siu, 2000). This is a serious issue for healthcare planners, administrators, and providers alike.

Barriers to adequate pain control in patients with dementia are multifold and include: limited ability to communicate, presence of multiple pain problems, increased sensitivity to drug side effects, and lack of physician education in regard to pain management. The consequences of inadequate pain control include: sleep disturbances, behavioral problems, decreased socialization, depression, impaired ambulation, and increased health care use and costs (Ferrell, 1995; Parmelee *et al.*, 1991).

In studies until comparatively recently only 1% of patients receiving hospice services had dementia as the primary diagnosis whereas 80% pf patients receiving hospice services had a diagnosis of cancer, reflecting the misconception that dementia is not a terminal illness. The PEACE program (Palliative Excellence in Alzheimer Care Efforts) was developed with the mission of moving palliative care "upstream", that is to integrate palliative care into the primary care of patients with dementia. Data were collected on 150, predominately African-American patient caregiver dyads and initial feedback by patients and families indicated high rates of satisfaction with the quality of care, adequate pain control, and appropriate attention to prior stated wishes. Two-thirds of the deaths occurred at home, the desired site for most patients known to have a preference (Diwwan *et al.*, 2004).

Findings from the PEACE program reinforce the idea that effective palliative care for dementia patients must address the various sources and types of caregiver strain and stress, provide adequate support to caregivers for the management of problem behavior, and offer counseling to help them families cope with the emotional challenge presented by the progression of dementia (Dwain *et al.*, 2004).

1. Conclusion

We have explored the complex array of palliative care issues that arise for families and physicians as AD progresses in this chapter. The functional impairments, personality changes and behavioral disturbances associated with AD are extremely burdensome for caregivers physically, emotionally, and financially. The burden may be diminished and nursing home placement may be delayed with continuous support and respite programs.

It is of crucial importance that physicians discuss the goals of care with both caregivers and patients. Physicians should emphasize the appropriateness of a focus on comfort when the disease is in its advanced stages. We are suggesting that medical testing and interventions should only occur if it is likely that they will result in improved quality of life. Hospital admissions and antibiotic use should be minimized and a "Do Not Resuscitate" order is recommended. Families need to be alerted to the fact that feeding tubes do not prevent aspiration pneumonia and are likely to have a negative impact on quality of life.

While medical testing and interventions are of questionable usefulness, we cannot overemphasize the importance of pain medication. Additionally, patients with AD should be referred to hospice relatively early, and not just in the last few weeks of life. While optimal care for AD patients and their families is extremely time consuming, when the suffering of patients is minimized their families and physicians are much more likely to be pleased with both treatments and outcomes.

References

Ahronheim, J.C., Morrison, R.S., Baskin, S.A., Morris J., and Meier D.E. (1996). Treatment of the Dying in the acute care hospital; advanced dementia and metastatic cancer. *Archives of Internal Medicine.* 156(18):2094-2100.

Ahronheim, J.C. (1996) Nutrition and hydration in the terminal patient. *Clinics in Geriatrics.* 12(2):379-391.

American Psychiatric Association. (1994). *Diagnostic and Statistical Manual of Mental Disorders, 4th ed.* Washington, DC: American Psychiatric Association.

Applebaum, G.E., King, J.E., and Finucane, T.E. (1990). The Outcomes of CPR Initiated in Nursing Homes. *Journal of the American Geriatric Society.* 38(3):197-200.

Cohen, C.A., Gold, D.P., Shulman, K.I., Wortley, J.T., McDonald, G., and Wargon, M. (1993). Factors determining the decision to institutionalize dementing individuals: a prospective study. *Gerontologist.* 33(6):714-720.

Cummings, J.L. Alzheimer's disease. (2004). *New England Journal of Medicine.* 351(1):56-67.

Diekema, D.J., BootsMiller, B.J., Vaughn, T.E., Woolson, R.F., Yankey, J.W., Ernst E.J., Flach, S.D., Ward, M.M., Francicus, C.L., Pfaller, M.A., and Doebbeling, B.N. (2004). Antimicrobial resistance trends and outbreak frequency in United States hospitals. *Clinical Infectious Diseases.* 38(1):78-85.

Fabiszewski, K.J., Volicer, B., and Colicer, L. (1990). Effect of antibiotic treatment on outcome of fevers in institutionalize Alzheimer patients. *Journal of the American Medical Association.* 263:3168-72.

Ferrell, B.A., Ferrell, B.R., and Rivera, L. (1995a). Pain in cognitively impaired nursing home patients. *Journal of Pain and Symptom Management.* 10(8):591-98.

Ferrell, B.A. (1995b) Pain evaluation and management in the nursing home. *Annals of Internal Medicine.* 123(9):681-87.

Finucane, T.E. and Bynum, J.P. (1996). Use of tube feeding to prevent aspiration pneumonia. *Lancet.* 348 (9039):1421-24.

Finucane, T.E., Christmas, C., and Travis, K. (1999). Tube feeding in patients with advanced dementia. *Journal of the American Medical Association.* 282(14):1365-1370.

Fried, T.R., Gillick, M.R., and Lipsitz, L.A. (1997). Short-term functional outcomes of long-term care residents with pneumonia treated with and without hospital transfer. *Journal of the American Geriatric Society.* 45(3):302-6.

Hanrahan, P. and Luchins, D.J. (1995). Feasible criteria for enrolling end-stage dementia patients in home hospice care. *Hospice Journal.* 10:47-54.

Hanrahan, P., Raymond, M., McGowan, E., and Luchins, D.J. (1999). Criteria for enrolling patients in hospice: a replication. *American Journal of Hospice and Palliative Care.* 16(1):395-400.

Head, B. (2003). Palliative Care for Persons with Dementia. *Home Healthcare Nurse,* Volume 21. Lippincott Williams and Wilkins, Inc., New York, pp. 53-61.

Hebert, L.E., Scherr, P.A., Bienias, J.L., Bennett, D.A., and Evans, D.A. (2003). Alzheimer disease in the US population: prevalence estimates using the 2000 census. *Archives of Neurology.* 60(8):1119-22.

Heyman, A., Peterson B., Fillenbaum, G., and Pieper, C. (1997). Predictors of time to institutionalization in patients with Alzheimer's disease. The CERAD Experience, Part XVII. *Neurology*. 48(5):1304-1309.

Kuebler, K.K., Lynn, J., and Von Rohen, J. (2005). Perspectives in palliative care. *Seminars in Oncology Nursing*. 21(1):2-10.

Luchins, D.J., Hanrahan, P., and Murphy, K. (1997). Criteria for enrolling dementia patients in hospice. *Journal of the American Geriatric Society*. 45(9):1054-1059.

Lunney, J.R., Lynn, J., Foley, D.J., Lipson, S., and Guralnik, J.M. (2003). Patterns of functional decline at the end of life. *Journal of the American Medical Association*. 289(18):2387-2392.

Marshal, G.A., Fairbanks, Telcin, S., Vinters, H.V., and Cummings, J.L. (2006). Neuropathologic correlates ofd activities of daily living in Alzheimer disease. *Alzeihmer Disease and Associated Disorders*, Jan-Mar: 20(1):56-9.

Mittelman, M., Ferris, S.H., Shulman, E., Steinberg, G., and Levin, B. (1996). A family intervention to delay nursing home placement of patients with Alzheimer's disease. *Journal of the American Medical Association*. 276(21):1725-1731.

Molsa, PK., Marttila, R.J., and Rinne, U.K. (1986). Survival and cause of death in Alzheimer's disease and multi-infarct dementia. *Acta Neurologica Scandanavica*. 74(2):103-7.

Morley, J.E. (2002). Orexigenic and anabolic agents. *Clinics in Geriatric Medicine*. 18(4):853-66.

Morris, J.C. (2003). Dementia Update 2003. *Alzeihmer Disease and Associated Disorders*. 17(4):245-258.

Morrison, R.S., Ahronheim, J.C., Morrison, G.R., Darling, E., Baskin, S.A, Morris J., Choi, C., and Meier, D.E. (1998). Pain and discomfort associated with common hospital procedures and experiences. *Journal of Pain and Symptom Management*. 15(2):91-101.

Morrison, R.S. and Siu, A.L. (2000). A Comparison of Pain and Its Treatment in Advanced dementia and cognitively intact patients with hip fracture. *Journal of Pain and Symptom Management*. 19(4):240-8.

Muder, R.R., Brennen, C., Swenson, D.L., and Wagener, M. (1996). Pneumonia in a long-term care facility: a prospective study of outcome. *Archives of Internal Medicine*. 156(20):2365-2370.

Odle, T.G. (2003). Alzheimer disease and other dementias. *Radiologic Technology*. 75(2):111-1135.

Parmelee, P.A., Katz, I.R., and Lawton, M.P. (1991). The relation of pain to depression among institutionalized aged. *Journal of Gerontology*. 46(1):15-21.

Porsteinsson, A.P., Tariot, P.N., Erb, R., Cox, C., Smith, E., Jakimovich, L., Noviasky, J., Kowalski, N., Holt, C.J., and Irvine, C. (2001). Placebo-controlled study of divalproex sodium for agitation in dementia. *American Journal of Geriatric Psychiatry*. 9(1):58-66.

Purtilo, R.B. and Have, A.M.J. (2004). Preface. In: Purtilo, R.B., Have, A.M.J. (eds.), *Ethical Foundations of Palliative Care for Alzheimer Disease*, John Hopkins University Press, Baltimore, p. V.

Rahkonen, T., Eloniemi-Sulkava, U., Rissanen, S., Vatanen, A., Viramo, P., and Sulkava, R. (2003). Dementia with Lewy bodies according to the consensus criteria in a general population aged 75 years or older. *Journal of Neurology, Neurosurgery and Psychiatry*. 74(6):720-4.

Reisberg, B. (1988). Functional assessment staging (FAST). *Psychopharmacology Bulletin.* 24(4):653-659.

Shadlen, M.F. and Larson, E.B. (2004). Diagnosis of Dementia. *Up to Date.* 12:3.

Stuart, B., Herbst, L., and Kinzbrunner, B. (1998). National Hospice Organization,. Hospice Care: A Physician's Guide. Published by National Hospice and Palliative Care Organization, Arlington, VA, 1998.

Volicer, B.J., Hurley, A. Fabiszewski, K.J., Montgomery, P., and Volicer, L. (1993). Predicting short-term survival for patients with advanced Alzheimer's disease. *Journal of the American Geriatric Society.* 41(5):535-40.

Volicer, L., Mckee, A., and Hewitt, S. (2001). Dementia. *Neurol Clin.* 19:867-885.

Volicer, L. (2001). Management of severe Alzheimer's disease and end-of-life issues. *Clinics in Geriatric Medicine.* 17(2):377-91.

10
Children and Issues Around Palliative Care

Tamara Vesel MD, Rita Fountain,
and Joanne Wolfe MD MPH*

1. Introduction

In 1993, Pediatric Palliative Care (PCC) was defined by the World Health Organization (WHO) as compassionate and all-inclusive care when curative treatment is no longer possible. Since then however, PCC has broadened into family-centered care aimed at enhancing quality of life and minimizing suffering of all children with life-threatening conditions, no matter what the outcome of the illness (Field and Behrman, 2003). As described by the American Academy of Pediatrics (AAP, 2000), the goal of PCC is to add life to the child's years, not simply years to the child's life.

Each year in the United States, approximately 50,000 children die and 500,000 children live with life-threatening conditions (Himelstein *et al.*, 2004). According to the 2002 Annual Summary of Vital Statistics (Arias *et al.*, 2002), 27,567 infants and 25,845 children and adolescents (1 to 19 years) died. Out of 53,455 total childhood deaths, 36% of children died from preventable injuries (Figure 10.1), suggesting that the bereavement needs of the surviving family, friends and community are vast. However, the majority childhood deaths are related to an unavoidable underlying chronic illness or condition (Figure 10.1; Feudtner *et al.*, 2002) and this is where palliative care strategies can make an enormous difference. A recent analysis of deaths of individuals less than 25 years old in Washington State found that 52 percent occurred in the hospital, 8 percent in the emergency department or during transport, and 22 percent at other sites, and 17 percent at home (Feudtner *et al.*, 2002).

TAMARA VESEL • Instructor in Pediatrics, Harvard Medical School, Attending Physician, Pediatric Advanced Care Team, Dana-Farber Cancer Institute and Children's Hospital Boston, 44 Binney Street, Boston, MA 02115. RITA FOUNTAIN • Coordinator, Pediatric Advanced Care Team, Dana-Farber Cancer Institute and Children's Hospital Boston, 44 Binney Street, Boston, MA 02115. JOANNE WOLFE • Assistant Professor of Pediatrics, Harvard Medical School, Director, Pediatric Advanced Care Team, Dana-Farber Cancer Institute and Children's Hospital Boston, 44 Binney Street, Boston, MA 02115 and *Corresponding author: Assistant Professor of Pediatrics Harvard Medical School, Director, Pediatric Advanced Care Team, Dana-Farber Cancer Institute and Children's Hospital Boston, 44 Binney Street, Boston, MA 02115.

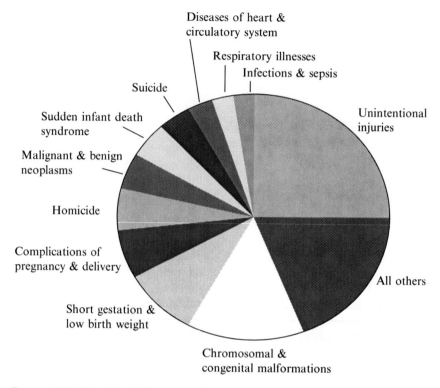

FIGURE 10.1. Diversity of illnesses and conditions leading to death in childhood.

In examining the trajectories of childhood death we can begin to determine the needs of children with life-threatening conditions and their families (Field and Cassel, 1997) (Figure 10.2). As noted, many children die suddenly and unexpectedly from unintentional injuries, homicide, and suicide (Figure 10.2A). Others may experience a steady and fairly predictable decline (Figure 10.2B), such as the child with a Tay Sachs disease. However the majority of children with life-threatening conditions will experience varying periods of chronic illness punctuated by crises, one of which may prove fatal (Figure 10.2C). Illnesses and conditions that typically follow this course include multiply relapsed cancer, cystic fibrosis, children with profound neurological impairment, advanced HIV and many others.

Thus, for most children with life-threatening conditions, the best approach to their care is one that blends interventions aimed at treating the underlying disease with those aimed at meeting the physical, psychosocial, and spiritual needs of the child and family (Sahler et al., 2000) (Figure 10.3). This approach turns out to be one that is favored by most parents, hoping for life-extension at the same time as maximal comfort for the child (Wolfe et al., 2000). In order to fulfill such hopes, optimal care of children with life-threatening

A. Sudden Death from an Unexpected Cause

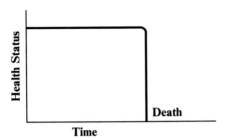

B. Steady Decline from a Progressive Disease with a "Terminal" Phase

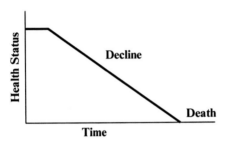

C. Advanced Illness Marked by Slow Decline with Periodic Crises and "Sudden" Death

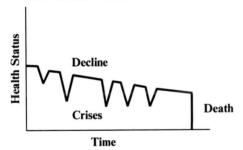

FIGURE 10.2. Prototypical death trajectories. **A:** Sudden death from an unexpected cause. **B:** Steady decline from a progressive disease with a "terminal" phase. **C:** Advanced illness marked by slow decline with periodic crises and "sudden" death. [Adapted from Field MJ, Cassel CK, Institute of Medicine (U.S.). Committee on Care at the End of Life. Approaching death: improving care at the end of life. Washington, D.C.: National Academy Press, 1997:29.]

conditions should include open communication, intensive symptom management, timely access to interdisciplinary care, which can be delivered in a flexible manner to meet the unique needs of an individual child and family. This model of care is both child and family oriented, with the ultimate goal of allowing for meaningful experiences.

Hope for cure, life extension, a miracle...

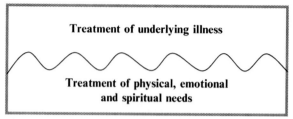

Hope for comfort, quality of life, meaning...

FIGURE 10.3. Blending of goals in caring for children with life-threatening illness and their families. [Adapted from Sahler OJ, Frager G, Levetown M, *et al.* Medical education about end-of-life care in the pediatric setting: principles, challenges, and opportunities. Pediatrics 2000;105:575–584.]

2. Barriers to Pediatric Palliative Care

In examining the scope of PPC, the complexity of needs becomes immediately apparent (Graham *et al.*, In Press) (Figure 10.4). Achieving the best possible care of children with life-threatening illnesses and their families requires an approach that encompasses all the elements delineated in the figure. More specific barriers are listed in Table 10.1.

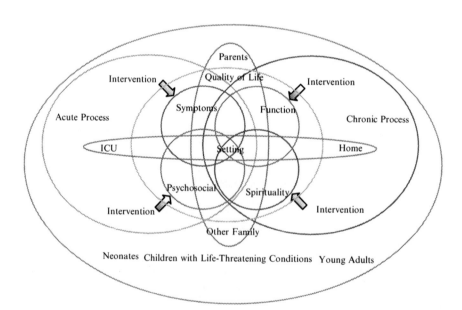

FIGURE 10.4. The scope of pediatric palliative care.
Source: Graham R, Dussel V, Wolfe J. Research in palliative care. In: Hain R, Goldman A, Liben S, eds. *Textbook of Pediatric Palliative Care*. Oxford: Oxford University Press; 2006.

TABLE 10.1. Barriers to optimizing pediatric palliative care and resulting consequences

General barriers	Consequence
Emotional considerations	Avoidance
Defiance of the natural order when children die	
Provider sense of failure when a child dies	
Immeasurable parental distress at loss of child	
Prognostic uncertainty	Delayed focus on palliative care
Rarity of death in childhood	Inexperienced providers
Diversity of childhood illness	Inexperienced providers
Little formal education of caregivers	Inexperienced providers
Poor reimbursement for time and labor-intensive, bio-behavioral palliative care	Under provision of services
Lack of developmentally appropriate assessment tools	Poor assessment and palliation of symptoms
Lack of pharmacokinetic data for children taking symptom relieving medications	Poor palliation of symptoms
Community Barriers	
Geographic diversity	Under serviced populations
Lack of universal healthcare coverage for all children	Lack of access to palliative care
Lack of reimbursement for critical services	Under provision of services
Hospice specific limitations	
Requirement of life-expectancy less than six months	Delayed involvement of hospice
Lack of experienced pediatric clinicians	Inexperienced providers
Daily reimbursement rates are low ($120/day)	Under provision of palliative care
Cannot be accessed if "extended hour nursing" already supports the child at home	Under provision of palliative care
Hospital Barriers	
May require emergency department visit	Disruption in continuity of care
Caregiver team	
New, less familiar	Poor assessment and palliation
Varying levels of experience	Inexperienced providers
Frequent changes	Poor assessment and palliation
Differing values	Under provision of services
Stay may be prolonged	Added cost
Care may be intensive even if patient has declined intensive care	Added cost

Emerging data suggests that, related to these barriers, there are areas in need of considerable improvement in the care of children with life-threatening conditions. Specifically, the data suggest that communication is suboptimal (Wolfe *et al.*, 2000; Kreicbergs *et al.*, 2004; Contro *et al.*, 2002) and that children experience substantial distress from symptoms at the end of life (Drake and Collins, 2003; McCallum *et al.*, 2000; Wolfe *et al.*, 2000). In response to the challenges in providing pediatric palliative care, the Institute of Medicine (IOM) recently released a report with sweeping recommendations for change related to

- Providing and organizing child- and family-centered care,
- Financing restructuring,
- Enhancing education of healthcare professionals,
- Research efforts focusing on improving the collection of descriptive data, and spanning the entire disease trajectory (Field and Behrman, 2003).

3. Models of Pediatric Palliative Care

There are emerging models of PPC that are striving to overcome the barriers as highlighted in Table 10.1, while incorporating well-considered IOM recommendations. What unifies these programs is the shared vision of providing comprehensive palliative care to children while optimizing the use of local expertise and resources. Since there are no current reimbursement mechanisms to support necessary palliative care services, all are partially to completely dependent on funding sources outside of currently available healthcare reimbursement, including institutional support, grants, congressional appropriations for demonstration models, and philanthropy. What follows are brief descriptions of several new models of PPC programs.

3.1. Children's Hospice International Program for All-Inclusive Care for Children and Their Families®

Children's Hospice International (CHI), a non profit organization founded in 1983 to provide a network of support and care for children with life-threatening conditions and their families, developed the Program for All-Inclusive Care for Children and their Families® (CHI PACC®), a model based on anticipated changes in regulation and reimbursement (http://www.chionline. org/programs/.). CHI PACC® demonstration projects have been developed in over 7 states through congressional appropriations and with technical assistance from Centers for Medicare and Medicaid Services using several Medicaid waiver options to support care services for seriously ill children. Unlike traditional hospice/palliative care models, a CHI PACC® program provides a continuum of care for children and their families from time of diagnosis, with hope for a cure, and through bereavement if a cure is not attained. Evaluation of the impact of these programs is ongoing.

3.2. The Seattle Pediatric Palliative Care Project

In 1998 a model demonstration program of PCC was implemented at Children's Hospital and Regional Medical Center in Seattle, Washington, to test an approach to PCC that embodied the principles of PCC practice: 1) family-centered ethical decision-making to elicit patient and family preferences; 2) provider training to promote improved communication, advance care planning, and shared decision-making; and 3) flexible administration of health plan benefits to support comprehensive and co-mingled curative and palliative interventions. The Seattle Pediatric Palliative Care Project (SPPCP) targeted children with potentially life-limiting illnesses in the state of Washington. It was supported by a three-year grant from the Robert Wood Johnson Foundation's program *Promoting Excellence in End of Life Care* from October 1998 through September of 2001. This model of care is based on unique contractual arrangements with local payers that allow reimbursement for expert care coordination and case management for children. The service negotiates with health plans to provide case management and to creatively administer benefits to meet individual needs. Central to accessing this model of individualized care is the Decision-Making Tool (DMT). The DMT is a process that improves communication among health care professionals and patients and families. The Palliative Care Consultants facilitate family-centered "DMT" care planning meetings with the patient, family and care team from all disciplines, including hospital staff, community care providers, and state agency and school personnel. These meetings provide opportunities to clarify treatment options and decisions, address advance care planning and anticipatory grief issues, and identify and strategize for community supports and services. The Palliative Care Consultants also provide professional support and education to hospital staff and other health professionals.

3.3. The Initiative for Pediatric Palliative Care

The numbers of hospital-based PCC programs are not known, however based on a survey of the National Association of Children's Hospitals and Related Institutions (NACHRI) the majority of hospitals do not offer specialized PCC. The Initiative for Pediatric Palliative Care (IPPC) was begun with the principal goal of developing a PCC curriculum and to support hospital-based quality improvement efforts aimed at enhancing family-centered care for children living with life-threatening conditions. IPPC's curriculum is complete and offers a comprehensive, interdisciplinary curriculum that addresses knowledge, attitudes and skills that health care professionals need in order to better serve children and families. With regard to quality improvement efforts, IPPC worked in collaboration with several national organizations, including NACHRI, along with seven children's hospitals to promote quality improvement projects aimed at improving palliative care for children.

Preliminary evidence suggests that improved outcomes are possible when PPC services are involved in the care of children with advanced illness. For example, in an age and diagnosis matched case-control study, Pierucci and colleagues demonstrated that infants receiving palliative care services were less likely to undergo interventions such as intubations and blood draws and were more likely to have social and chaplaincy services involved in their care (Pierucci et al., 2001). Preliminary data from Hamel and colleagues also found that with the advent of a PPC service at the Dana-Farber Cancer Institute and Children's Hospital Boston, parents of children who died of cancer were more likely to report that their child experienced significantly less suffering from symptoms and, overall, they were more prepared for the child's end-of-life course as compared to historical controls (Hammel et al., 2001).

At the Children's Hospital Boston and the Dana-Farber Cancer Institute this PCC service, the Pediatric Advanced Care Team (PACT), has been supporting children with life-threatening conditions and their families since 1997. PACT participated in the IPPC initiative with the goal of serving more children with non-oncological diagnoses. This quality improvement effort was very successful, and now approximately two thirds of PACT patients have diagnoses other than cancer. The following two cases from the PACT experience highlight some of the barriers to good quality palliative care for children with life-threatening illness discussed previously, and show how children with life-threatening conditions and their families can be better served.

4. Overcoming Community Barriers to Delivering Optimal PCC

James was an 11 year-old cheerful boy with multiple congenital anomalies including a complex congenital heart disease due to chromosomal abnormalities. He underwent multiple surgical procedures during his life, which required numerous lengthy hospitalizations. By the time James was 9-years old, his parents and older siblings came to a mutual decision about future goals of care. They wanted James to continue to be able to maintain a happy, pain-free life that avoided trips to the emergency department (ED) or physician's office, and for James to spend quality time with his family and teachers. He and his family lived two hours from his usual healthcare facility. James' family members felt strongly about their desire to limit his exposure to medical facilities, and any invasive procedures that would not enhance his quality of life. At that time, he was enrolled in a local hospice. However, approximately one year later due to his continued longevity and with no change in his underlying life-limiting condition, he was discharged from hospice and instead received approval for 100 hours per week of nursing support at home. Unfortunately, nursing resources were far more limited and approved nursing hours could not be filled.

Regrettably, this family could not achieve their goals for James because the medical system was unable to support complex decision-making from a distance. When changes in James' condition developed, his parents were directed to the local ED (where there was limited expertise and resulting discomfort addressing the medical issue at hand) or they were asked to return to the outpatient clinic for direct assessment even though they lived two hours away. The family felt misunderstood and not well supported in their goals and asked for the involvement of the PACT. After a phone conversation with the family, the palliative care team set up a home visit. Shortly after this initial consult at their home, James developed aspiration pneumonia. His family still wanted James to remain at home and again requested assistance with symptom management. Since his pediatrician did not feel comfortable providing complex medical care at home, the family contacted PACT again. The PACT re-involved hospice and when James continued to deteriorate, they supported the hospice nurse via phone to augment her comfort with pediatric end of life care. PACT clinicians coordinated communication with the family, home nurses, pediatrician, and hospice nurses throughout the remaining days of his life. James died in the arms of his family, surrounded by nursing staff and a hospice nurse in his favorite room overlooking the birdfeeders in the garden.

James' story illustrates numerous barriers that are present in our current health care system when managing a child with a progressive complex medical condition from a distance. Despite the parents' effort to plan James' care well in advance, the health care system was not able to match their needs. Continuous communication and support of the families' goals was fragmented due to the shift between various organizations and caregivers, e.g.; transition home, discharge from hospice care. This fragmentation complicates communication and the family is forced to explain their wishes repeatedly. A palliative care service helps to bridge the gap by providing longer-term continuity, helping the family feel understood and reassuring them in their decision-making.

The extreme complexity of this child's medical condition mandated that the family train the home nurses in James' specialized care in order to avoid a 2-hour drive to a tertiary care center which clearly disrupted their lives. They faced this challenge again when James was in the last stages of his life. However, this time the challenge was overcome through the combined care by hospice and the tertiary care PPC team. This benefited James and directly matched the families' overall goal to keep James at home with maximum comfort.

Despite the support of a PCC, there remained barriers to optimal care of James and his family. Ideally, there should be no limit to the duration of involvement of hospice in the care of a child with a life-threatening illness. As illustrated in Figure 10.2C, the gradual decline of the child with increasing possibility of dying suggests the high likelihood of hospice re-involvement in the future. In this case, hospice became re-involved 3 days prior to the death of James and there was only limited time for preparing the family. Eligibility requirements for hospice should be more flexible for children with advanced illnesses and there is a need for further development of PCC services in order to bridge the support from the hospital to the home.

Pediatric hospice expertise was also extremely limited. In accordance with ChIPPS, 2001, of the 3,000-plus existing hospice programs in the US, only 450 reported that they were prepared to provide hospice services to children (CCsPopH, 2001). Though exact numbers are not known, it is estimated that there are fewer than 100 pediatric hospice programs in the United States (Field and Behrman, 2003). The programs that have been successful longer term have done so in partnership with large adult hospice programs and/or through extensive philanthropic support. Even fewer programs offer residential services for children. Finally, additional education in symptom management could be beneficial to pediatricians and home care staff (Hilden et al., 2001).

5. Overcoming Hospital Barriers to Delivering Optimal PCC

Jacob was a 6.5-month-old sweet baby boy, who was born with severe perinatal encephalopathy of unclear origin. He remained on a life support machine (ventilator) for his first week of life until his family decided to withdraw the ventilator due to the poor prognosis. Jacob was able to breath on his own but was unable to suck or swallow. His parents were told that he needed to receive nutrition via a nasogastric tube and after proper training they were discharged home. At the time, the parents understood that Jacob's life would be significantly shortened.

Jacob's parents sought the support of the PACT to help them with their decision making regarding Jacob's quality of life. The following month Jacob required treatment for a complicated seizure disorder and despite maximum medical management began experiencing a lot of discomfort during and after feeds. At the same time, his parents were striving to normalize his life despite his complex medical care. They actively participated in extended family activities, continued to travel, and enjoyed their son. The last two weeks of Jacob's life were spent at the hospital after he was admitted due to increase in pain and discomfort. He underwent a trial of nasojejunal feeds but remained extremely uncomfortable while being fed. After multiple conversations with his parents it became evident that they felt his suffering and poor quality of life were unbearable and were not consistent with their hopes.

When the option of surgical intervention to provide nutrition was presented to the family, they shifted their goals for Jacob. Because the PACT had been involved in their life continuously over several months, they openly discussed their thoughts about withdrawal of fluid and nutrition. After numerous discussions they asked the PPC team to share their thoughts with their interdisciplinary health care team who agreed that withdrawing nutrition would be appropriate for Jacob. The parents invited their extended family and community clergy to come to the hospital to share their decision about Jacob in a meeting facilitated by the PACT. The child and family were moved to a home-like suite in the hospital, which enables the family to be together with their child and loved ones in a more comfortable setting. Jacob received medication for seizures and other symptom relief and died comfortably in the arms of his parents.

Jacob's story illustrates how early involvement of palliative care services can help to overcome multiple barriers that arise in the hospital when making difficult decisions for infants and children with severe life-limiting conditions. Primary care pediatricians may be unfamiliar or uncomfortable with counseling or managing a child with life-threatening illness, given the rarity of a child's death in a pediatric practice (McGrath and Finley, 1996). This is where the early involvement of the PACT directly impacted Jacob's family and their decision making process. The earlier this relationship begins, the more likely it is to be helpful. The PACT spent numerous sessions talking with the family about Jacob's quality of life and assisted in the exploration of their hopes and values, religious beliefs, and philosophical outlook on life. This enabled the parents to share their deepest feelings about Jacob's suffering and his inability to enjoy a basic life necessity as food. The PACT was then able to share Jacob's family's hopes and goals with the rest of the medical team, avoiding conflict with caregivers who were less familiar with them, and who may have had varying levels of experience and differing values. Not every family will be able to openly plan for their child's end-of-life experience, however a long-term relationship with a PPC can lead to easier implementation of palliative care plans when the time is right. The home-like suite allowed Jacob and his parents to be together in a supportive environment with expertise in palliative and end-of-life care close at hand.

6. Conclusion

There are emerging models of care aiming to better meet the needs of children with advanced illness, their families, and communities. However, these are few in number and outcome data are limited. Though the numbers of affected children are small, there exists a societal obligation to this vulnerable patient population to provide comprehensive, interdisciplinary and compassionate care. Beyond the individual child, the health of parents, healthy siblings and community members is also at stake long-term. High quality PPC is simply as expected standard. Through further quality improvement and formal research endeavors we need to determine the best ways to meet this standard.

References

American Academy of Pediatrics. (2000). Committee on Bioethics and Committee on Hospital Care. Palliative care for children. *Pediatrics*. 106(2 Pt 1):351-357.

Arias E., MacDorman M.F., Strobino D.M., Guyer B. (2003). Annual summary of vital statistics–2002. *Pediatrics*. 112(6 Pt 1):1215-1230.

Contro N, Larson J, Scofield S, Sourkes B, Cohen H. (2002). Family perspectives on the quality of pediatric palliative care. *Archives of Pediatric and Adolescent Medicine*. 156:14-19.

Drake RFJ, Frost J, Collins JJ. (2003). The symptoms of dying children. *Journal of Pain and Symptom Management*. 26(1):594-603.

Field MJ, Behrman RE. (2003). Institute of Medicine (U.S.). Committee on Palliative and End-of-Life Care for Children and Their Families. *When children die : improving palliative and end-of-life care for children and their families*. Washington, D.C.: National Academy Press.

Feudtner C, Christakis DA, Connell FA. (2000). Pediatric deaths attributable to complex chronic conditions: a population-based study of Washington State, 1980-1997. *Pediatrics*. 106(1 Pt 2):205-209.

Feudtner C, Silveira MJ, Christakis DA. (2002). Where do children with complex chronic conditions die? Patterns in Washington State, 1980-1998. *Pediatrics*. 109(4):656-660.

Field MJ, Cassel CK. (1997). Institute of Medicine (U.S.). Committee on Care at the End of Life. *Approaching death: improving care at the end of life*. Washington, D.C.: National Academy Press.

Graham R, Dussel V, Wolfe J. (2006). Research in palliative care. In: Hain R, Goldman A, Liben S, eds. *Oxford Textbook of Palliative Care for Children*. Oxford: Oxford University Press.

Hammel JF, Klar N, Comeau M, et al. Improved satisfaction regarding end-of-life care among parents of children with cancer related to implementation of a palliative care service. Paper presented at: Proc. Pediatric Academic Societies, 2001.

Hilden JM, Emanuel EJ, Fairclough DL, et al. Attitudes and practices among pediatric oncologists regarding end-of-life care: results of the 1998 american society of clinical oncology survey. *Journal of Clinical Oncology*. 2001;19(1):205-212.

Himelstein BP, Hilden JM, Boldt AM, Weissman D. (2004). Pediatric palliative care. *New England Journal of Medicine*. 350(17):1752-1762.

Kreicbergs U, Valdimarsdottir U, Onelov E, Henter JI, Steineck G. (2004). Talking about death with children who have severe malignant disease. *New England Journal of Medicine*. 351(12):1175-1186.

McGrath PJ, Finley GA. (1996). Attitudes and beliefs about medication and pain management in children. *Journal of Palliative Care*. 12(3):46-50.

McCallum DE, Byrne P, Bruera E. (2000). How children die in hospital. *Journal of Pain & Symptom Management*. 20(6):417-423.

Pierucci RL, Kirby RS, Leuthner SR. (2001). End-of-life care for neonates and infants: the experience and effects of a palliative care consultation service. *Pediatrics*. 108(3):653-660.

Program for All-Inclusive Care for Children and their Families (CHI PACC). htt://www.chionline.org/programs/

Sahler OJ, Frager G, Levetown M, Cohn FG, Lipson MA. (2000). Medical education about end-of-life care in the pediatric setting: principles, challenges, and opportunities. *Pediatrics*. 105(3 Pt 1):575-584.

Children's Project on Palliative/Hospice Services (CHIPPS). (2001). *A call for Change: Recommendations to Improve the Care of Children Living with Life-Threatening Conditions*. Alexandria, VA: National Hospice and Palliative Care Organization. www.NHPCO.org (chipps@nhpco.org).

Wolfe J, Klar N, Grier HE, Duncan J, Salem-Schatz S, Emmanuel EJ, Weeks JC. (2000). Understanding of prognosis among parents of children who died of cancer: impact on treatment goals and integration of palliative care. *Journal of the American Medical Association*. 284(19):2469-2475.

Wolfe J, Grier HE, Klar N, Levin SB, Ellenbogen JM, Salem-Schatz S, Emmanuel EJ, Weeks JC. (2000). Symptoms and suffering at the end of life in children with cancer. *New England Journal of Medicine*. 342(5):326-333.

11
Palliative Care and the Elderly: Complex Case Management

Sean O'Mahony MB BCh BAO, and Franca
Martino-Starvaggi CSW

1. Introduction

The number of chronically ill and disabled elderly people with complex medical, psychosocial and financial needs is rapidly growing. The elderly population has been steadily increasing in the United States due to the efforts of modern medicine and disease prevention techniques. The elderly will now live for three to six years prior to death with increasing levels of disability (Fried, 2002).

The US health-service was designed several decades ago when life expectancy was shorter and the duration of disability before death was brief. Its emphasis on curative and disease focused interventions is poorly aligned with the complex healthcare needs of the elderly and their caregivers. Shorter lengths of stay in acute care hospitals and limitations in eligibility to even the most basic levels of homecare render frail elderly patients more susceptible to the complications of multiple competing chronic illnesses. Increased disability, poly-pharmacy, strained resources and caregiver systems, limited knowledge and precarious decisional capacity are complications not addressed by traditional models of health-service, thus resulting in episodic, unplanned delivery of service and preventable hospitalizations with a focus on individual diagnoses.

In order that elderly patients may be better served, complex case management models will need to be integrated into primary care delivery and specialty palliative care programs across multiple healthcare settings. In this chapter we will describe the demographic data that support the development of such models and some of the key elements that are integral to the provision of case management to elderly patients at the end-of-life.

SEAN O'MAHONY • Palliative Care Service, Department of Family and Social Medicine, Montefiore Medical Center, Albert Einstein College of Medicine, Bronx, NY, USA, 111 E. 210th Street, Bronx 10467. • FRANCA MARTINO-STARVAGGI • Montefiore Medical Center, Palliative Care Service, Department of Family and Social Medicine, Bronx, NY.

2. The Demography of Ageing in the United States

The percentage of the population over the age of sixty-five years has been projected to grow from 12% in 1984 to an expected 22% in 2050 with the fastest growing segment comprised of those over the age of eighty-five years (Briar and Kaplan, 1990). As the elderly live longer, so do their children and there is recognition that soon the elderly will be the caregivers of the older elder population. Thirty-five percent of caregivers are currently over the age of sixty-five and 10% are over seventy five years of age and many of them are female (Clark and Weber, 1997). Dependency is also expected to vary by gender. Women who are sixty-five years old are expected to live to eighty-four years of age, fourteen of those years can be expected to be active, five years dependent. Men at sixty-five can expect fifteen more years of life, twelve years of which will be fully independent. Nonetheless, at age eighty-five, nearly half of the remaining years will be dependent (Kahn et al., 2000). Functional dependence is not the only change evident with increased longevity. The dysregulated immune system that occurs in the aged may account for the pathogenesis of some age-specific disorders including cancer, alzheimer's disease, and osteoporosis (Thoman and Weigle, 1981). Regardless of what changes occur, the elderly will be affected by multiple problems including medical issues, the environment, personal support system, limited finances and reduced capacity for decision-making.

3. Functional Ability

Medical problems present a particular hardship when they occur in the aged. The Hospital Outcomes Project for the Elderly (HOPE), a prospective study of 1279 community-dwelling elderly patients who were hospitalized for acute medical conditions evaluated functional and other outcomes. Among those who declined in function, 40% declined in three or more activities of daily living (ADL). For patients at 3 months after discharge, 19% reported new ADL disabilities (Margitic et al., 1993). Probably the most predictable source of functional loss is that due to immobility. In elderly patients there is rapid deconditioning in response to even short periods of bed rest. Decline in mobility occurs with varying degrees in the elderly who are hospitalized, studies indicate that 15-60% of elderly who are hospitalized become dependent in activities such as ambulation, transfers and toileting (Hirsch et al., 1990; Mahoney et al., 1998). The elderly are more susceptible to worsening disability in response to hospitalization and chronic illnesses and subsequent institutionalization than younger adults (Sharma et al., 2001; Kaye et al., 1996; Manton et al., 1993).

4. Poly-pharmacy and Falls

Nocturia, anemia, stroke, emphysema, cancer, cataracts, and glaucoma are some of the more common co-morbidities associated with increased risk of falls in the elderly (Herndon *et al.*, 1997; Stewart *et al.*, 1992; Cumming, 1998).

Similarly, the elderly are the most vulnerable segment of the population to the impact of poly-pharmacy. The average ambulatory elderly patient has 11 prescriptions filled yearly and eight medications are prescribed for the average nursing home resident. Data from the 1994 National Hospital Ambulatory Medical Care Survey revealed that potentially inappropriate medications were prescribed at 4.5% of outpatient visits by elderly patients (Aparasu and Sitzman, 1999). The most common adverse drug reactions in elderly patients involve the genitourinary and psychiatric/central nervous systems (Klein *et al.*, 1984). Adverse drug reactions may often appear as a worsening medical condition in a demented patient, or falls in an already unsteady patient. Elderly patients at the end-of-life face pain and many other symptoms which compound functional deficits. In addition pain and other symptoms are under-medicated and commonly not assessed in the elderly (Von Roenn *et al.*, 1994; Bernabei *et al.*, 1998; Desbeins *et al.*, 1996).

Older adults taking more than three or four medications are at risk for recurrent falls (Leipzig *et al.*, 1999). In addition, some studies have found a relationship between the usage of non-steroidal anti-inflammatory drugs with falls (Field *et al.*, 1999).

5. The Social World of the Elderly

The living environment is another area that affects the elderly. Extremes in temperatures render them at risk of dehydration, electrolyte abnormalities such as hypernatremia (increased sodium concentration in the blood) and rhabdomyolysis (muscle breakdown which may occur as a result of dehydration). They may be unable to sustain their socialization and some of their instrumental activities of daily living such as getting to places beyond walking distance and grocery shopping (Lawton and Brody, 1969). Limited transportation results in increased isolation and reduced access to care.

Support systems affect the elderly as they become more dependent on other people, especially their family. The number of available caregivers is shrinking. More female caregivers are now working and they are usually the caregivers of the elderly. Family caregivers often do not live close to their elderly parents. The number of paid caregivers will also continue to decline as the population continues to age. They are currently amongst the lowest paid workers in our society. They often work without health care benefits or paid vacation and lack opportunities for the development of their skills.

Unsurprisingly, attrition rates are very high for this segment of the work force: disproportionately women of color and immigrants.

The financial situation of the elderly is one of the more complex issues they face. They are no longer employed, dependent on a fixed income and any saved assets. In the U.S., the American Association of Retired Persons reports that only 40% of patients older than 75 have prescription coverage, in contrast to 75% of those in the 45 to 54 age brackets (AARP, 1996). The inflation of rent, property taxes and increased cost of utilities, food and medicine often result in choosing between purchasing medications, food, or traveling costs to their monthly medical appointments. Even minor reductions in prescription coverage for elders with limited resources have been demonstrated to be associated with increased rates of institutionalization.

(Soumari *et al.*, 1987; Dannis *et al.*, 1997; Cole *et al.*, 2006; Kronish *et al.*, 2006; Mojtabi and Olson, 2003).

6. Decision Making for the Elderly

The capacity for decision-making is an important factor in the care of the elderly. Kennedy (2000) speaks at length about capacity in the elderly. His principles are outlined below.

6.1. Principles of Decisional Capacity Assessment

- Competence and capacity are used interchangeably, but it is capacity that is the issue in clinical settings. Capacity may fluctuate but still be adequate. Decisional capacity is specific to circumstances.
- The adequacy of capacity depends on an understanding of the risks, benefits, and burdens of proposed intervention and the consequences of the specific choice.
- People who have decisional capacity should be able to understand that they are being asked to make a choice and express the choice consistently.
- Appreciate the nature of their condition including diagnosis, prognosis, and possible treatments.
- Balance the risks, benefits, and burdens of various choices.
- Apply a relatively stable set of values to the choice of available options.
- Communicate the rationale behind the choices.

People with decisional capacity who are aware of the consequences of their choices should be allowed to assume the resultant risks. Evaluation by a psychiatrist is advisable when decisional capacity is in question. When patients lack capacity, they should be protected from the consequences of impaired decisions. When capacity is indeterminate, other factors external to the patient are given consideration (e.g. caregivers and family). When the patient has capacity but makes an unwise decision, there may still be areas of agreement that support a collaborative, albeit less than optimal, plan of care with health care providers. The exercise of poor judgment is not synonymous with impaired capacity.

7. Hospital, Home Care, Nursing Homes and Hospices

In addition to the multiplicity of personal issues which affect the elderly, the health care systems with which the elderly interface are quite limiting to their needs at times. Hospitals have changed tremendously over the last fifteen years due to the rising costs of healthcare. Elderly patients who were hospitalized in the past were never discharged until they had fully recovered from their medical illness. If they felt too weak to go home, they remained in the hospital until they were stronger. This is no longer the case. Patients including the elderly are expeditiously sent home and much of the time they have not fully recovered. Early analysis suggested that Medicare beneficiaries were indeed being discharged "quicker and sicker" and in more unstable condition, but no effect on 30- day or 6- month mortality could be readily identified (Kahn et al., 1990; Kosecoff et al., 1990).

As a result of the decreasing length of hospital stay, nursing homes have changed as well. Nursing homes are now used as an intermediate place for elderly people to fully recover from their hospitalization. Recovery in the nursing home is severely time constrained because it will only be covered by most medical insurances for twenty days.

Homecare is another healthcare system that has limitations for the elderly., Access to paid homecare has become more restricted since the Balanced Budget Act in 1997. For example, Medicare will only pay for patients who have an acute skilled need, leaving a large group of frail elderly people who have multiple chronic medical problems less able to get any form of homecare services at all. Medicare regulations for homecare will be discussed in greater detail later on in the chapter. Medicaid rarely provides coverage for twenty-four hour home attendants. As a result, patients who require round the clock care are often forced to go into nursing homes rather than be able to remain in their home environment.

Hospice is another system that some elderly people interface with at some point at the end of their life. Older adults with advanced dementia or end stage cardiac disease tend to have a high burden of co-morbidities and functional limitations; therefore, they are usually in need of more custodial care. Due to the financial limitations of the hospice benefit, elderly patients with limited financial means who may need more personal care services may be unable to get their needs adequately met in hospice. For elderly patients with limited means who are not yet dually eligible for Medicaid and Medicare hospice care in a skilled nursing facility may also not be an affordable option, as the patient will be required to pay for "room and board" in the facility.

7.1. Limitations of the Medical Model

A pure primary medical model often has limitations for geriatric patients. Geriatric practices tend to have a team-based focus which includes geriatricians, nurses, social workers, dieticians, physical and occupational therapists. These disciplines tend to bring in other perspectives that are not disease-specific, but focus more on function and social aspects of the elderly. In primary care settings, there often isn't such a team approach. The physician's evaluation is disease-based as opposed to function-based and may not provide the complete picture of the elderly patient. It has also been suggested in the literature that primary care physicians find elderly patients more difficult to treat (Damiano et al., 1997; Adams et al., 2002).

8. Pulling It Together: Palliative Care

The formalization of advance directives is of central importance to case management in the elderly. Sudden catastrophic illness or slowly progressive disease may make it impossible for elderly people to communicate their wishes. Advance directives may help preserve the autonomy of the elderly and may make their wishes known when they can no longer communicate. Advance directives are usually formalized with the assistance of physicians and hospital personnel when a medical crisis occurs. There continue to be deficits in the discussion of advance directives with seniors by both family members and physicians. Even if elderly patients have previously executed directives, they are often ignored or not documented on medical records and often poorly predictive of the type of care that a patient may receive. Instead there may be a reliance on surrogates and physicians recollection of patient wishes which maybe poorly correlated with the wishes of elder patients. Older adults with impaired functional status when presented with hypothetical scenarios in which life prolonging treatments are warranted often opt in favor of these interventions at least for time-limited trials. Elderly patients' interpretation of their quality-of-life is not necessarily reflective of current functional status or co-morbid conditions. Despite this, physicians commonly invoke quality-of-life as an argument against the use of life prolonging treatments in the elderly (Shmerling et al., 1988; Hammes and Rooney, 1988; Uhlmann et al., 1988; Hamel et al., 1989; Torian et al., 1992; Quill and Bennett, 1992; Morrison et al., 1995; Dannis et al., 1997; Murphy and Santilli, 1998; O'Mahony et al., 2003).

Besides decisions regarding medical treatment options, important decisions must be made about personal and individual financial planning. The elderly often prefer to make these decisions on their own rather than to "burden" their family/friends by having them assist them. When the elderly are faced with making decisions in a hospital setting, practitioners tend to include their family and/or surrogate in this process. Communication and education are of vital importance in assisting all involved in making these decisions. The more information they have regarding their medical options and the clearer the information that is presented to them, the easier it will be to make an educated choice.

9. Managing Complexity: Case Management and Palliative Care

Case management facilitates positive outcomes for the elderly. It is defined by the American Nurses Association (1991) as a healthcare delivery process that provides quality healthcare, decreases fragmentation, enhances the client's quality-of-life, and contains costs. Homebound elderly who receive case management services experience fewer hospitalizations and have lower healthcare costs (Burns *et al.*, 1996).

Many issues are balanced and incorporated in making plans for and with the elderly population. They include: medical insurance and resources, identification and involvement of the family support system, assessment of the functional and decisional capacity of the elderly person, cultural values assessment, and previously expressed wishes of an incapacitated person, or if the person has capacity, the expressed wishes of the individual. Finally, the medical teams' viewpoints, pre-conceived notions and their backgrounds are also fundamental in making case management decisions for the elderly. These issues need to be all equally considered in order for the plan to be successful. Lack of a complete and comprehensive assessment, will hinder the outcome of the plan of care.

1. *Medical insurance and resources is usually addressed first.* Adequate health insurance of the elderly person and his financial resources will determine all other available options, since it is quite clear that these define the power to purchase whatever is needed to fulfill their needs.

Every person over the age of sixty-five years who was born in the United States and who has worked for ten years in this country automatically receives Medicare insurance. The federal government made Medicare available in 1966 and it is the major payer for home health care. In the 1970s, the Medicare benefit was expanded to include persons under the age of sixty-five who were disabled and or chronically ill for the past two years. Medicare covers some of the costs of inpatient hospitalization, inpatient and outpatient physician services, diagnostic tests, and procedures. If a person is hospitalized and needs rehabilitation Medicare will pay for approximately twenty days in a skilled nursing facility. If one needs homecare services, Medicare insurance will pay for a registered nurse, physical therapist and/or speech therapist to go into their home only if there is a skilled need that can be fulfilled in the home. The person also has to be home-bound. Medicare coverage for homecare was originally intended for short-term, post-acute care. A person may have numerous chronic medical problems and may need assistance in self caring, but this is not considered a skilled need nor is it a basis for Medicare to pay for services in the home. In New York City for example home health aide coverage is limited to approximately twenty hours a week and when there is no longer a skilled need to monitor or be taught by the nurse, the nurse and the home health aide will be required to withdraw from providing services. In Texas, the average amount of personal care or home health care services is as little as three hours a week.

Managed insurance payers tend to follow similar guidelines to Medicare in terms of homecare services and nursing home coverage, but they are more stringent than Medicare and they do not provide as extensive benefits or care. The freedom to choose physicians, hospitals, homecare agencies and nursing homes is removed, but the enrollees have fewer out-of-pocket expenses in return.

Eligibility for Medicaid, a state administered federally funded health insurance, on the other hand, is based on the person's financial resources. Eligibility requirements for Medicaid and the amount of care that it affords vary widely from state to state. In New York City in 2005, for a one person household, the maximum monthly income is $667.00 and the person should have less than $5,550.00 in resources including a $1,500 burial fund, as well as their own home and car. If a person is Medicaid eligible, they are able to go into a nursing home if medically necessary and it will be paid for the rest of their life. If the person needs extended homecare services regardless of whether or not they have a skilled need for a nurse, they can also receive this for the rest of their lives providing they are safe in the community and there are formal or informal supports supervising the care.

2. *The support system is the second most important issue to evaluate for formulating plans.* As a person becomes more frail and more dependent on others, it is important to assess who is the significant support system for the elderly person and how involved they are able or willing to be for the elderly person. In making case management decisions, if an elderly person wants to remain in their home environment, it is imperative that there are family members who live close by and are able to commit to visiting frequently to supervise the care or provide direct care. Families who work full time, have their own nuclear family obligations or have their own medical problems are already often unable to add more responsibilities to their already stressful lives. If an elderly person lacks an adequate support system, then it is much more difficult for an elderly person to reside in the community with a palliative care plan.

3. *The component of capacity assessment of the elderly person is the next issue that is crucial in case management.* As mentioned before, capacity for decision-making whether it be for health care or advance care planning is based on whether the person is able to receive the information, evaluate, mentally manipulate the information as well as to communicate a preference in a logical manner. By the same token, if the person no longer has the capacity, but their support system is aware of the previously expressed wishes, it may be just as valuable as if the person had the ability to express their wishes at

the present time. The socially-isolated elderly person who has no capacity is the most vulnerable particularly if he has no health care proxy, living will or advance directives. Medical staff will treat the individual as if he has agreed to aggressive medical treatment and consent for tests or procedures must be provide by the administrative staff. More complicated or risky treatment will require the facility's administration to involve the judicial system. A court appointed guardian can make decisions in regard to either the patient's financial affairs or medical care. This is usually done as a last resort as it is quite costly and it takes approximately six months before it is processed.

4. *The functional ability of the elderly person is the next issue to be addressed.* Elderly people with fewer chronic illnesses and greater functional integrity are more likely to remain in the home environment and continue to be independent in response to intercurrent acute illnesses. As the patient becomes more dependent on others and has more medical problems warranting more skilled nursing care, it becomes increasingly challenging for the person to remain in the community.

5. *Culture, ethnicity and religion play a major role in case management of the elderly.* Certain cultures are expected to care for their elderly family members in the home until the end of the elder's life and other cultures do not feel the same obligation. When one is assessing and making plans for an elderly person, it is critical to know and understand their religious and cultural background, so that one can appreciate where their decisions are rooted. On the other hand, it is imperative not to make generalizations based on ethnicity and religion. Treating an individual as if they are their own "race, ethnicity and religion" is the best approach when making an assessment.

6. *The final issue to be addressed which is perhaps one of the most problematic is the medical team's viewpoints, preconceived notions and their backgrounds when making case management decisions with the elderly.* The team approach is a critical element in working in a hospital setting. The team approach gives greater objectivity in discerning treatment goals, "sharing the burden" of medically complicated patients, increased clarity of one's role and increased awareness and respect for the other disciplines. There is also improved access to care for patients and their families. It can be quite difficult at times to incorporate all of the various viewpoints and backgrounds and make decisions that everyone is in agreement with. The team's role is to educate and inform the patient and their surrogate of the medical issues so that they can make their own informed decisions.

10. Case Studies of Complex Case Management in Palliative Care

The following are some examples of case management with the elderly which will illustrate all the issues discussed and how they are incorporated within an assessment.

10.1. Case Study 1

Ms. CD is a 75-year-old Irish single roman catholic female who was admitted to the intensive care unit from a local nursing home. She was admitted with respiratory failure, and had a history of alzheimer's dementia, coronary artery disease, and hypertension. The patient is dependent on a ventilator. Ms. CD has a gastric feeding tube for nutrition and hydration. Due to her immobility, she has sacral ulcers. The patient is responsive to touch and needs complete care. The patient has been a resident of a local nursing home for the last two years.

The patient's sole support system is her older widowed sister, Mrs. ED. Both sisters lived together for most of their lives. When the patient's father was dying, he told Mrs. ED to take care of her younger sister. Mrs. ED took these "words to heart". She kept her sister at home for as long as possible but reluctantly placed her in a nursing home two years ago. The patient never made any advance cares plans (neither living will nor a health care proxy). When the physicians approached the patient's sister regarding a "do-not resuscitate" order, she adamantly refused. Mrs. ED wanted the patient to be treated aggressively in all treatment plans regardless, of the medical team's evaluation of her prognosis as being poor. Initially, Mrs. ED presented as a regressed and mentally limited individual, yet the substance of her conversations adequately related to the medical issues being addressed. She was persistent, and vocal in making her sister's needs known and was often suspicious and distrustful of the staff and team. She was truly her advocate, yet it was unclear if this was actually representative of the known wishes of the patient. She had never appointed a health care proxy, yet her sister was her only support system. One has to also take into account the religious upbringing of the D's, which was clearly significant in the decisions as well. She was a devout roman catholic and would often be observed to be saying the rosary in the patient's room.

The outcome of this difficult and emotional case was that the team did aggressively treat Ms. CD in deference to the wishes of Mrs. ED. There came a point however in the patient's care at which the antibiotics were no longer effective. The team finally set limits and told Mrs. ED that there was no more that could be done for her in terms of antibiotic therapy and she was sent to a new ventilator nursing home facility that Mrs. ED had chosen.

Mrs. ED felt somewhat comfortable and content with the fact that her sister did get all the care possible, yet she still wanted her sister cured and was resistant to accepting that this would never be a reality. There are often only certain amounts of information that family members can truly understand and accept and then an impasse is reached, and it can be unrealistic to expect the family members to cross that impasse.

10.2. Case Study 2

Mrs. CG is a 77- year-old widowed african american female who was admitted to a geriatric inpatient medical unit. Her diagnoses included chronic venous insufficiency, infected bilateral leg ulcers, diet-controlled diabetes mellitus, and mild dementia. Her wounds were so severe that they were foul smelling with areas of moist necrotic tissues, surrounded by peeled tissue and bleeding. She had three previous hospitalizations related to her noncompliance in her treatment and further deterioration of her bilateral leg ulcers.

She was alert and oriented, with periods of confusion and usually able to make her needs known. Mrs. CG did not participate in any activities of daily living except feeding herself when her meal was set-up by the nursing staff. She would refuse to have the nurse do daily wound dressing changes. Due to her unwillingness to accept treatment, medically speaking, her prognosis was poor. When questioned about her compliance, she never had any clear answers. She would either say, "Not today", "I'm tired." or "leave me alone." Throughout her hospital stay, the patient was verbally abusive to staff. She would also throw her meal tray at the nursing staff out of anger and hostility. She wanted to return home with 24-hour care when she was medically stable for discharge.

She lived alone in a fifth floor walk-up apartment. She was known to two home health agencies and she had received twelve hours/7 days a week home health aide services for the past two years. She had "fired" over twenty-five home attendants in the previous two years.

Mrs. CG had one daughter who occasionally stayed with the patient. She had a history of alcohol abuse, verbal and physical abuse of the nurses and the home health aides, as well as financial abuse of Mrs. CG. Adult Protective Services (APS) became involved prior to the patient's admission to begin guardianship proceedings, to protect the patient from the daughter's financial abuse as well as the patients' poor judgment and lack of insight.

Mrs. CG had another daughter (R.C.) who visited the mother at home and in the hospital sporadically. RC had five children for whom she cared on a daily basis. She claimed she was unaware of her sister's abuse towards her mother. She was angry with the team for not having her mother go home with twenty-four hour care. She could not accept or understand that no agency would accept Mrs. CG into their program again. RC finally accepted her mother would not receive any formal home care services unless she paid privately for them or she could take her mother home in her care, however, she was unwilling to do either. She subsequently agreed to nursing home placement for her mother as well as becoming her court-appointed guardian.

Mrs. CG never appointed a health care proxy, because she did not trust anyone to make decisions for her, except herself. She also refused to have any discussions regarding advance directives. Mrs. CG wish to be treated aggressively was evidenced by statements that she wanted "everything done", yet she wouldn't participate in her daily active treatment. She refused to sign do-not-resuscitate orders, because she felt then her doctors would let her die and not care for her any longer.

CG had mild dementia and two geriatric psychiatrists felt she did not have capacity to make decisions. CG, however, was quite verbal and capable of directing her care and making decisions- even if they weren't the best decisions to make. The team wanted her to listen to their judgment and follow the treatment plan. The team wanted to protect her and place her in a safe environment.

The goals of care of the team and of CG were in direct contrast necessitating the appointment of a guardian. The team wanted her to be treated appropriately, cooperate in the treatment, and be in a safe environment. CG's goals of care were to be allowed to do whatever she wanted and to be home with twenty-four hour care.

The resolution of CG and the team's conflict was acheived during the guardianship proceedings. The judge's decision was two-part. He felt the team should attempt to have her go home in the care of her daughter and an older cousin who presented for the first time at the guardianship proceedings. The judge felt that the hospital should instruct them on proper care and supervise this care for the patient within the hospital for two weeks. If they were successful, CG could go home even though she did not have capacity to make decisions.

During this two-week time period, RC only came twice and the cousin stayed at the hospital for forty-eight hours. After forty-eight hours, she never came back to the hospital, nor did the team hear from her again. The judge then decided on placement for CG in a skilled nursing facility that RC had selected and she was appointed guardian. CG remained in the nursing home for a little over two years and then died in the nursing home.

11. Conclusion

The demographic changes that are occurring currently and which will continue in the coming decades in part relate to advances in medical technologies; ironically the multiplicity of problems and chronic co-morbidities that occur in the frail elderly also highlight the limits of these technologies. The unplanned requirement for life prolonging therapies in response to the inevitable progression of an individual illness may result in short term improvement in one condition; but ultimately other illnesses become more prominent and each individual episode of acute illness is accompanied by greater levels of disability with a return to a previous baseline level of functioning becoming progressively more remote. Financial resources are depleted and familial caregiver resources are stretched even further. The demographic shifts that we have described ultimately will create leverage for the creation of medical systems that integrate case management into the scope of practice of all medical, social work and nursing specialties and will create a healthcare system that must be responsive to the multiple domains of need for this population.

References

Adams, W.L., McIlvain, H.E., Lacy, N.L., Magsi, H., Crabtree, B.F., Yenny, S.K., and Sitorius, M.A. (2002). Primary care for the elderly people: why do doctors find it so hard? *The Gerontologist*. 42:835-842.

American Association for Retired People. (1996). Older people are pinched by drug costs. *AARP Bull* 33:3.

American Nurses Association (1991). Nursing's agenda for healthcare reform.

Aparasu, R.R. (1999). Visits to office-based physicians in the United States for medication-related morbidity. *Journal of the American Pharmaceutical Association (Wash.)*. May-June; 39(3):332-337.

Bernabei, R., Gambassi, I., and Lapane, K.F. (1998). Pain management in elderly patients with cancer. *Journal of the American Medical Association*. 279(23):1877-82.

Briar, K.H. and Kaplan, C. (1990). The family caregiving crisis. Silver Spring, MD: National Association of Social Workers.

Burns, L.E., Lamb, G.S., & Wholey, D.R. (1996). Impact of integrated community nursing services on hospital utilization and costs in a Medicare risk plan. *Inquiry*. 33: 30-41.

Clark, J.A. & Weber, K.A. (1997). Challenges & choices: family relationships- elderly caregiving Missouri: University of Missouri-Columbia.

Cole, J.A., Norman, H., Weatherby, L.B., and Walker, A.M. (2006). Drug copayment and adherence in chronic heart failure: effect on cost and outcomes. *Pharmacotherapy*. 26(8):1157-64.

Cumming, R.G. (1998). Epidemiology of medication -related falls and fractures in the elderly. *Drugs Aging*. 12(1):43-53.

Damiano, P., Momany, E., Willard, J., and Hansen, C. (1997). Factors affecting primary care physician participation in Medicare. *Medical Care*. 35:1008-1019.

Dannis, M., Biddle, A.K., Henderson, G., Garrett, J.M., and DeVellis, R.F. (1997). Older Medicare enrolees' choices for insured services. *Journal of the American Geriatric Society*. 45(6):688-694.

Desbiens, N.A., Wu, A.W., Broste, S.K., Wenger, N.S., Connors, A.F. Jr., Lynn, J., Yasui, Y., Phillips, R.S., and Fulkerson, W. (1996). Pain and satisfaction with pain control in seriously hospitalized adults: Findings from the SUPPORT research investigations. *Critical Care Medicine*. 24(12):1953-61.

Field. T.S., Gurwitz, J.H., Glynn, R.J., Salive, M.E., Galiano, J.M., Taylor, J.O., and Hennekens C.H. (1999). The renal effects of nonsteroidal anti-inflammatory drugs in older people: findings from the Established Populations for Epidemiologic Studies of the Elderly. *Journal of the American Geriatric Society*. 47(5):507-11.

Fried, L.P. (2002) epidemiology of aging. *Epidemiologic Reviews* 22 (1):95-106.

Hammes, B.J., Rooney, B.L. (1998). Death and end-of-life planning in one Midwestern community. *Archives of Internal Medicine*. 158(4):383-390.

Hamel, M.B., Teno, J.M., Goldman, L., Lynn, J., Davis, R.B., Galanos A.N., Desbiens N., Connors, A.F., Wenger, N., Phillips, R.S. (1999). Patient age and decisions to withhold life sustaining treatments from seriously ill, hospitalized adults *Annals of Internal Medicine*. 130:116-125.

Herndon, J.G., Helmick, C.G., Sattin, R.W., Stevens, J.A., DeVito C., Wingo P.A. (1997). Chronic medical conditions and risk of fall injury events at home in older adults. *Journal of the American Geriatric Society*. 45(6):739-743.

Hirsch, C.H., Sommers, L., Olsen, A., Mullen, L., and Winograd, C.H. (1990). The natural history of functional morbidity in hospitalized older adults. *Journal of the American Geriatric Society*. 38 (12):1296-1303.

Kahn, K.L., Kieler, E.B., Sherwood, M.J., Rogers, H., Draper, D., Bentow, S.S., Reinisch E.J., Rubenstein, L.V., Kosecoff, J., and Brook, R.H. (1990). Comparing outcomes of care before and after implementation of the drg- based prospective payment system. *Journal of the American Medical Association*. 264(15):1984-1988.

Kaye, S., LaPlante, M.P., Carlson, D., and Wenger, B.L. (1996). Trends in disability rates in the United States, 1970-1994. National Institute on Disability and

Rehabilitation research report. Washington DC: US. Department of Health and Human Services. Available online at http://dsc.ucsf.edu/UCSF/pub

Kennedy, G.J. (2000). *Geriatric Mental Health Care.* Guilford Press, New York.

Klein, L.E., German, P.S., Levine, D.M., Feroli, E.R. Jr., and Ardery, J. (1984). Medication problems among outptients. *Archives of Internal Medicine.* 144:1185-1188.

Kosecoff, J., Kahn, K.L., Rogers, W.H., Reinisch, E.J., Sherwood, M.J., Rubenstein, L.V., Draper, D., Roth, C.P., Chew, C., and Brook, R.H. (1990). Prospective payment system and impairment at discharge. *Journal of the American Medical Association.* 264(15):1980-1983.

Kronish, I.M, Federman, A.D., Morrison, R.S., and Boal, J. (2006) Older Medicare enrolees' choices for insured services. *The Journals of Gerontology Biological Sciences and Medical Sciences.* 61(4):411-5.

Lawton, M.P. and Brody, E.M. (1969). Assessment of older people: self-maintaining and instrumental activities of daily living. *The Gerontologist.* 9:179-186.

Leipzig, R.M., Cumming, R.G., Tinetti, M.E. (1999). Drugs and falls in older people: a systematic review and meta-analysis: I. Psychotropic Drugs. *Journal of the American Geriatric Society.* 47(1):30-39.

Mahoney, J.E., Sager, M.A., and Jalaluddin, M. (1998). New walking dependence associated with hospitalization for acute medical illness: Incidence and significance. *The Journals of Gerontology Biological Sciences and Medical Sciences.* 53:307-312.

Manton, K.G., Corder, L.S., and Stallard, E. (1993). Estimates of change in chronic disability and institutional incidence and prevalence rates in the US elderly population from the 1982, 1984 and 1989 National Long Term Care Survey. *Journals of Gerontology Psychological Sciences and Social Sciences.* 48:S153-166.

Margitic, S.E., Inouye, S.K., Thomas, J.L., Cassel, C.K, Regenstreif, D.I, and Kowal, J. (1993). Hospital outcomes project for the elderly (HOPE): Rationale and design for a prospective pooled analysis. *Journals of the American Geriatric Society.* 41(3): 258-267.

Mojtabi, R. and Olson, M. (2003). Medication costs, adherence, and health outcomes among Medicare beneficiaries. *Health Affairs (Millwood).* 22(4):220-229.

Morrison, R.S., Olson, E., Mertz, K.R., and Meier, D.E. (1995). The inaccessibility of advance directives on transfer from ambulatory to acute care settings. *Journal of the American Medical Association* 274(6):478-482.

Murphy, D.J., and Santilli S. Elderly patients' preferences for life-support (1998). *Archives of Family Medicine* 7:484-488.

O'Mahony, S., McHugh, M., Zallman, L., Selwyn, P. (2003). Ventilator Withdrawal: Procedures and outcomes, a retrospective review of a collaboration between a critical care division and palliative care service: *Journal of Pain and Symptom Management.* 26(4):954-961.

Quill, T.E., and Bennett, N.M. (1992). The effects of a hospital policy and state leglislation on, resuscitation orders for geriatric patients. *Archives of Internal Medicine.* 152:569-572.

Sharma, R., Chan, L.H., and Ginsberg C. Health and health care of the Medicare population: data from the 1997 Medicare current beneficiary survey. Rockville MD: Weststat.

Shmerling, R.H., Bedell, S.E., Lilienfeld, A., and Delbanco, T.L. (1988). Discussing cardiopulmonary resuscitation. *Journal of General Internal Medicine.* 3:317-321.

Soumerai, S.B., Avorn, J., Ross Degnan, D., and Gortmaker, R. (1987). Payment restrictions for prescription medications under Medicaid. *New England Journal of Medicine.* 317(9):550-6.

Stewart, R.B.., Moore, M.T., May, F.E., Marks, R.G., and Hale, W.E. (1992) Nocturia: a risk factor for falls in the elderly. *Journal of the American Geriatric Society*. 40(12):1217-1220.

Thoman, W., and Weigle, W.O. (1981). Lymphokines and aging: interleukin-2 production and activity in aged animals. *Journal of Immunology*. 127:2102-2106.

Torian, L.C., Davidson, E.J., Fillit, H.M., Fulop, G., and Sell, L.L. (1992). Decisions for and against resuscitation in an acute geriatric medicine unit serving the frail elderly. *Archives of Internal Medicine*. 152:561-565.

Uhlmann, R.F., Pearlman, R.A., and Cain, K.C. (1988). Physicians' and spouses' predictions of elderly patients' resuscitation preferences. *Journal of Gereontology*. 43:M115-M121.

Von Roenn, J.H., Cleeland, C.S., Gonin, R., Edmonson, R.H., Blum, R.H., Stewart, J.A., and Pandya, K.J. (1994). Pain and its treatment in outpatients with metastatic cancer. *New England Journal of Medicine*. 330(9):592-6.

Wagner, A. (1984). Cardiopulmonary resuscitation in the aged. *New England Journal of Medicine*. 310(17):1129-1130.

12

The Business of Palliative Medicine: Business Planning, Models of Care and Program Development

Ruth Lagman MD MPH
and Declan Walsh* MSc FACP FRCP (Edin)

Abstract

Palliative Medicine is gradually being recognized as an invaluable clinical service. Currently there is a growing national interest to establish palliative medicine programs. A forward-looking, detailed business plan outlining the operational and financial projections over a period of time is key to the survival of a program. This chapter describes the business planning and program development implemented at the Cleveland Clinic, the first integrated and comprehensive palliative medicine program in the United States.

1. The Business Plan

1.1. Overview

A serious commitment to establish a palliative medicine program mandates that the process be conducted in a business like manner given the present health care environment. The goals of the program have to be specific and clearly defined and the process to realize these goals have to be outlined in detail. Therefore a comprehensive, forward-looking business plan written in the decision maker's language is imperative (Walsh *et al.*, 1994). When the program at the Cleveland Clinic set out their business plan in 1992, palliative medicine was a relatively (and still is) new concept in medical care that it was felt that it would be evaluated and judged more thoroughly compared to

RUTH LAGMAN • The Harry R. Horvitz Center for Palliative Medicine, Cleveland Clinic Taussig Cancer Center. DECLAN WALSH • Director, The Harry R. Horvitz Center for Palliative Medicine, The Cleveland Clinic Foundation, 9500 Euclid Avenue, M76, Cleveland, OH 44195 and *Corresponding author: Director, The Harry R. Horvitz Center for Palliative Medicine, The Cleveland Clinic Foundation, 9500 Euclid Avenue, M76, Cleveland, OH 44195. Tel: (216) 444-7793, fax: (216) 445-5090, e-mail: walsht@ccf.org existing traditional services. This reassured the senior administration at the institution that program development was serious, tangible and fiscally responsible. The program was able to meet its specific objectives that were realized in a timely fashion. These objectives were also in line with the overall goals of the Cleveland Clinic (Walsh, 2000).

The creation and subsequent implementation of a business plan requires a group of individuals with varying skill sets. At its inception, the group included the Director of the Palliative Care program, the Clinical Program Manager, the Nursing Director for Oncology Services, the Director of Business Development, Manager of Market Planning, Manager of Market Research, and a Fiscal Manager. Depending on the structure of a particular institution, the composition of the group may be revised.

1.2. Environmental Analysis

In creating an environmental analysis, it is important to identify strengths, weaknesses and opportunities that the program will encounter. The palliative medicine program at the Cleveland Clinic was the first of its kind to offer a comprehensive integrated palliative medicine program in 1987 and was designated a World Health Organization Demonstration Project in 1991 (Walsh, 2001). Since then, the interest to establish palliative medicine programs in the United States has grown exponentially as evidenced by the number of scientific meetings and the present number of fellowship programs in the country. The Medicare reimbursement system to palliative medicine has been favorable through the years. Given the limits of resources available, however, third party payors, both private and public, are looking for ways to best allocate resources to provide the best patient outcome outside of an acute care hospital setting. Because Medicare is the predominant payor for palliative medicine services, legislative changes in reimbursement and policy are a potential risk. However, even as there is a growing awareness of palliative medicine services, referrals to palliative medicine and hospice are still deferred until the final days of the patient's life. Enrollments have increased since 1992 but the median length of stay in hospice has decreased from 34 days to 22 days in 2003. 36.9% of those served by hospice died within seven days or less (National Hospice and Palliative Care Organization, 2003). This is significant because the stress on the professional caregiver staff is at the beginning and the end when the delivery of services is most intense.

1.3. Program Assessment and Development

Since the goal of a palliative medicine program is to be comprehensive and integrated it should offer a variety of services consisting of different product lines, i.e., clinical service areas that will allow patients to access each branch of service seamlessly while being cared for by one provider. By navigating through acute inpatient care, home hospice, inpatient hospice, home care, and outpatient clinic, overall costs should be lowered as continuity of care is provided by one dedicated multidisciplinary team (Walsh, 2001; Ahmedzai & Walsh, 2000; Tropiano & Walsh, 2000; Lagman & Walsh, in press; Melson & Walsh, 2005). The availability of a 24-hour emergency phone service to patients and families reduces their anxiety. Most questions and problems can be resolved over the phone. If indicated, admission to the hospital can be arranged directly while bypassing the emergency room. This again can help reduce costs and improve patient satisfaction by eliminating long waiting times.

Corollary to program development is the emphasis on research and education. The continued education of the professional caregivers (physicians, nurses, social workers) and the incorporation of a research program would allow patients and families access to new therapies and palliative interventions especially in an academic medical center (LeGrand et al., 2000).

1.4. Operational Needs

The multidisciplinary approach to caring for palliative medicine patients will require an increase in the number of health care professionals as the program grows. Being a comprehensive integrated program with different clinical service areas providing flexible access points to patients and families, it is then necessary to document the need for increasing staff.

1.5. Financial Feasibility

It is essential that a palliative medicine program be integrated and comprehensive to allow the program to be financially sound. A consultation or outpatient model alone may not be financially viable (Walsh, 2000). By offering a variety of services, i.e., acute inpatient medicine, home hospice, home care, inpatient hospice, outpatient clinic, and a 24-hour consultation service, several entry points to the program are identified. Individuals move from one service area to another depending on their specific needs. The advantage is that revenues earmarked for these services are kept within the program. Each can stand alone and is financially viable. More importantly, quality control over patient care is maintained as the program is integrated.

Because patients move from one service area to another, they are managed by one medical team who are familiar with the patient's medical and psychosocial history. Furthermore, the use of a formulary that is consistent within the integrated program allows medication costs to be contained. Medications that are administered in the acute inpatient palliative medicine unit are the same drugs that will be used in hospice. In the capitated reimbursement of hospice care in the United States, invasive palliative procedures are prohibitively expensive and that any of these procedures are done in an acute inpatient medical setting before transitioning to hospice.

It is important that palliative medicine take primary care on all patients. There are several advantages, namely 1) allow higher reimbursement rate because palliative medicine physicians are responsible for the day-to-day care of the patients, 2) specialty care is being given to this patient population, 3) allow access to different services of the program, 4) are judged by the same standards administratively as any other specialty (7).

1.6. The Role of Marketing

Palliative medicine patients eventually succumb to their advanced illness and that in order for the program to be sustainable, a constant stream of referral source for new patients have to be available. A marketing plan and strategy is a top priority in the program's growth strategy. It is important to identify opportunities and challenges in the prevailing health care market. These are key to formulating a marketing strategy.

Determining the growth in the cancer population over the next several years is important. If the palliative medicine program would treat and serve other individuals with non-malignant life-limiting illness, it is then important to seek out the growth of this patient population. The next important aspect to look at is payor source. With Medicare dominating the payor landscape because of the particular patient population being served, other opportunities for alternative payor source, i.e., managed care contracts, can be explored if the penetration is small.

Gathering patient outcomes and marketing favorable patient and family feedback regarding services rendered can be used as a marketing tool for the program. Given that most referrals come from within the Cleveland Clinic Health System, internal marketing to various physicians, nurses, case managers, and social workers will increase awareness of the program and hopefully generate more referrals.

1.7. Action Plan

After the business analysis, an action plan can be implemented. This includes 1) initiating a consult model palliative care program, developing an inpatient acute care unit, and hospice home care, 2) hiring well trained personnel as program growth is achieved and 3) implementing the proposed marketing plan (1).

1.8. Threats

There are several threats to establishing and maintaining a palliative care program. They are: 1) since Medicare is the major payor source for hospice and palliative medicine, changes in legislation regarding decreased reimbursement and delivery of care may impact the overall financial health of the program, 2) the shortages of well trained staff, i.e., nurses, physicians and

TABLE 12.1. Summary of services by year

Year	No. of consultations	Total inpatient admissions	No. of hospice admissions	Outpatient clinic visits
1988	323	7	N/A	N/A
1989	360	13	N/A	N/A
1990	379	269	7	N/A
1991	430	254	214	1,004
1992	477	316	272	956
1993	493	369	287	670
1994	568	476	274	910
1995	536	655	311	873
1996	744	722	488	1,316
1997	846	708	611	1,229
1998	843	633	672	1,374
1999	872	769	N/A	1,705
2000	1,065	823	624	N/A
2001	834	727	499	2,567
2002	984	821	676	1,716
2003	1,110	795	793	1,518
2004	1,173	892	761	1,444

N/A: Not Available

social workers specifically trained to do hospice and palliative medicine made worse by the high burnout rate in this field, 3) the continued source of new patient referrals to the program given the high turnover of patients.

1.9. Timelines and Milestones

The different clinical areas that the palliative medicine program currently offers has taken over 10 years to be developed, adding a new clinical service area approximately every 18 months (Walsh, 2000). It is a testament to the complexity and difficulty of developing a comprehensive and integrated palliative medicine program (See Table 12.1). The time and effort invested were utilized to demonstrate why each clinical service area was needed and how each can be financially viable. Presently, there is a current business plan in use for each clinical service area for operational and financial projections. This also includes a three-year time frame for added services in the future.

2. Program Development

2.1. Developing the Concept

Over the past decade, education, research and the media have focused on finding a cure for patients with advanced illness. Sadly, the reality is that the majority of these patients still die from their disease. Their clinical course is often laden with physical, psychosocial, spiritual and financial burdens. Death is inevitable and a comprehensive program must address the needs of this patient population (Walsh & Gordon, 2001; Sheehan & Twaddle, 2002). Compounding the problem is the rapidly aging population. It is estimated that by the year 2030, 64.3 million (21%) will join the ranks of the elderly (Tauber, 1893). They will develop some form of chronic illness, either malignant or non-malignant, demanding the same (or more) services that present individuals with advanced illness now need. In the United States, payments in the last year of life account for 27–30% of the total Medicare budget (Lubitz & Riley, 1993; Experton et al., 1996). Therefore, in establishing a palliative medicine program, desirable clinical outcomes include improvement in symptom control and patient satisfaction while reducing costs to the institution in terms of decreased length of stay and judicious use of hospital resources (Meier, 2002).

For all Americans who died in 2003, 50% died in an acute care setting, mostly with chronic advanced illness (National Hospice and Palliative Care Organization). This is a patient population that has always existed in acute care hospitals but whose needs were never clearly defined. The result has been disorganized, fragmented care. This is the target population that palliative medicine should focus on. Of note, in 1999, there were about 30% of institutions reporting hospital based palliative medicine programs with 42% of these based in large community hospitals and academic health centers (Pan et al., 2001).

2.2. Quality of Care

In establishing a palliative medicine program, a physician trained in palliative medicine is essential to the viability of the program. Doing so will bring a unique skill set necessary to provide comprehensive care to patients with advanced disease. These are: 1) communication, 2) symptom control, 3) management of complication, 4) care of the dying, 5) psychosocial care, and 6) coordination of care (17). It has been shown that integrating palliative medicine has actually improved the care of the terminally ill in acute care settings (Mandredi et al., 2002; Virik & Glare, 2002). The presence of a palliative medicine program can have several advantages to both patient care and the institution. They are: 1) providing clinical services in terms of symptom control, psychosocial care and discharge planning, 2) supporting other specialties in the institution in sharing the complex management of individuals with advanced illness, 3) allowing a system where the institution's goals can be accomplished (Glare et al., 2003).

The presence of specialist palliative care teams do improve outcomes for cancer patients. A systematic literature review that included five randomized controlled trials showed that patients and caregivers that were taken care of by palliative medicine specialists had improved symptom control, better satisfaction scores by patients and caregivers, decreased length of stay in hospital with a corresponding decrease in overall cost. In addition, patients were more likely to die in a place of their choice (Hearn & Higginson, 1998).

2.3. Understanding the Finances of Your Program

You are your own accountant. Understanding the financial details of your own palliative medicine program is important. Given the limited resources available for health care reimbursement, it is best to allocate these precious limited resources to services that will produce the best outcome. It is tempting to use philanthropic funds to cover operational shortfalls but this strategy is probably unwise. There is no guarantee that these funds will consistently be there. It is best to examine all aspects of the program and determine how costs can be contained instead and practice strict financial discipline.

2.4. Seek Out Your Strengths

The goal of a palliative medicine program is to meet the specific and unmet needs of individuals with advanced disease. It is essential that the program work with individuals who are strong advocates of the program. It is important that a palliative medicine program aligns its activities with the strategic goals of the organization, consult with institutional leadership on a regular basis to guide its activities and integrate existing clinical procedures and policies that the organization may have in place for oversight of care of the dying particularly in regard to the withdrawal of life prolonging therapies. Hence, in addition to providing quality service in the care of the dying, there is a need to solicit philanthropy and community support that can be used for future program development, and continuing education of the professional caregiver staff.

2.5. Avoidance

As with anything new, expect that there will be individuals who will be openly hostile to the program. It is important to focus limited energy and resources to the constructive and positive attributes of the program while not ignoring constructive criticism. It is also best to tune out negative attitudes about the program itself. It is vital that quality of care is served to the needs of this unique patient population. As the population served increases, the program will hopefully be able to sell itself even to those who were openly hostile from the beginning.

Though cost savings is one of the goals for establishing a palliative medicine program, it should not be the primary goal. It would be a tremendous risk for an institution to finance a new venture with no proven track record that may eventually lose money in the future. Furthermore, if the cost savings is not reached, the program may have doomed itself to perpetual downsizing. The key is to invest time and resources over a reasonable and realistic time frame while providing quality patient care (2). Examples of projected cost savings that some programs may include in their business plans include projections for reductions in hospital length of stay for specific diagnostic related groups, reductions in charges for diagnostic interventions in specific DRG's, charges for specific interventions such as ventilators in patients who die on their last hospitalizations, intensive care unit utilization and inter-unit transfers. Other potential measures of value to the organization include the proportion of patients dying within the medical center that receive service from a palliative care service as well as overall number of deaths within the setting of the medical center. If significant funding for a program is being solicited from managed care organizations potential options include projections for readmissions to acute care for specific DRG's (Smith *et al.*, 2004; O'Mahony *et al.*, 2005).

2.6. Marketing

When implementing the marketing program, it is important to have careful choice of words and titles. Talking about death is still taboo in the general population. Furthermore, misinformation about the dying process and the services available in caring for the dying is prevalent. Presently, palliative medicine is in itself evolving. The current experts in the area are in disagreement about definition and terms. Palliative care is the philosophy of caring for patients with advanced illness. Palliative medicine is a specialty discipline that sets standards on how to care for this unique patient population. It involves structured and formal fellowship training for physicians with board certification, formal training to nurses with certification and emphasis on education and research. Hospice, from which palliative medicine had its roots, has to be defined differently from palliative medicine. When palliative medicine/care is used synonymously and interchangeably with hospice, there will be confusion on what type of services is being provided. A subset of patients who are currently getting anti-tumor therapy may be well served by palliative medicine specialists when they are acutely ill but may choose not to come if the program is referred to as hospice (Davis *et al.*, 2002).

2.7. Clinical Care

The success of the program hinges on the delivery of care at the time it is requested. Hence, a multidisciplinary staff should be immediately available when the consult request is called. This ensures that the service is legitimate and not second rate. When the quality of service is recognized, this may be enough to change the mind of naysayers. The best advertisement to the program is the positive feedback from patients and families who benefited from the service. Also, since most patients have multiple distressing physical symptoms that need to be relieved, it is essential that these are evaluated and managed as soon as possible.

3. Structure of the Palliative Medicine Program

3.1. Consult Service

Palliative medicine as a service is a consult driven specialty. It is important that the stream of patient referral is constant given the limited life expectancy of this patient population. This has to be 24-hour, 7-day consult service as there is no predictability on when patients fall ill. Given this, a palliative medicine physician, trained and equipped with unique clinical skills is the cornerstone of the program (Lagman & Walsh, In Press). This physician should be supported by a multidisciplinary team, i.e., nurse clinician/practitioner or a physician extender and a social worker.

3.2. Acute Inpatient Unit

Most individuals with advanced illness are admitted emergently and need to be cared for by palliative medicine specialists and nurses. A specialized unit serving this patient population has several advantages; namely 1) palliative medicine physicians take primary over these patients and are reimbursed at a higher rate, 2) these same physicians have control over use of appropriate interventional and therapeutic interventions, 3) control access points to different aspects of the comprehensive program, 4) have input in the financial viability of the program. Since physicians are stationed in the unit most times, nurses can readily call for assistance in patient care. Moreover, physicians need not waste valuable time and energy walking around the institution to care for patients in a scattered bed model (7). Though the benefits are obvious, the financial outlay to establish a dedicated acute inpatient palliative medicine unit may be prohibitive but not impossible. The Cleveland Clinic was fortunate to have been given an endowment by the Harry R. Horvitz Foundation for the initial construction of the acute inpatient palliative medicine unit in 1994 (Goldstein et al., 1996). Since then the operations on the unit has been supported solely from revenues derived from patient care and has remained profitable (Davis et al., 2002; Davis et al., 2001). We have also identified a subset of the inpatient population at the Cleveland Clinic that would benefit from an acute care palliative medicine inpatient unit (Walsh, 2004).

3.3. Home Hospice and the Inpatient Hospice Unit

While majority of deaths still occur in an acute medical setting, only about 9% of hospice patients die in hospital (National Hospice and Palliative Care, 2003). As part of a comprehensive integrated program, patients can be cared for at home with hospice care. The advantage is that patients and families are in familiar surroundings and getting the benefit of a hospice nurse case manager overseeing his/her care. In addition, because hospice care is holistic in its approach, patients and families benefit from a multidisciplinary care team with physicians, nurses, social worker, pastoral care, and home health aides. Cost is also saved because patient is at home and not in an inpatient facility. The Cleveland Clinic decided to start its own hospice in the early part of the program development as there were concerns over the quality of care when this service was outsourced. Moreover, the palliative medicine program and the institution were losing revenues that it might have kept within the system instead. It is one of the few hospices in the United States owned by an academic medical center (Walsh, 2000).

As part of their hospice benefit, individuals can be admitted to an inpatient hospice unit for symptom management under the general inpatient level should more intense care be given than what can be provided for at home. The Hospice of the Cleveland Clinic operates its own 13-bed inpatient unit at the far west side of Cleveland. Bed space is also allotted for residential and respite care.

3.4. Home Care

Individuals who are currently undergoing active anti-tumor treatment but who may qualify for a skilled need may be eligible for home care. Examples of skilled needs are home physical therapy, home infusion with antibiotics or intravenous fluid, parenteral analgesia with a patient controlled analgesia (PCA) pumps for intrathecal/epidural catheter. Home care offers another access to the integrated comprehensive program as patients can be admitted to the inpatient unit for symptom management or they can have be transitioned to hospice once their anti-tumor therapies have been exhausted.

3.5. Outpatient Clinic

The outpatient clinic offers an opportunity for periodic follow-ups of patients and their physicians. Most are well enough to travel from home to the hospital. This offers another venue for new referrals. The outpatient clinic of the palliative medicine program runs in parallel to the hematology/oncology clinics. If possible, patients are seen on the same day by their oncologist and their respective palliative medicine physician. The early intervention of palliative medicine in the disease trajectory of individuals with advanced illness paves the way for a seamless model of eventually transitioning patients to palliative medicine (Cancer Pain Relief, 1990). New patient referrals are seen immediately because outpatient clinics run in parallel.

3.6. Nurse Case Management

Each individual patient is assigned to a palliative medicine physician who works in collaboration with a nurse clinician. The close contact and follow-up with the nurse clinician allows a relationship to develop. During office hours, patients can call in for questions regarding medications, symptoms and follow-up appointments. Most problems can be managed over the phone with medication adjustments. When symptoms become worse and an inpatient admission is warranted, the nurse can give the patient's respective physician an update and admission can be arranged promptly. An after-hours pager is available for calls from patients needing help during nights and weekends.

4. Other Models

The purpose and mission of a palliative medicine program will need to be tailored to the needs and mission of its respective institution. Most palliative medicine programs are hospital based because majority of adult deaths still occur in the acute care setting. The needs that are seen in these instances include: 1) addressing physical symptoms, 2) lack of communication about patients' goals of care, 3) lack of awareness of patient and family preferences, 4) financial, psychosocial, physical needs of caregivers, 5) high turnover of medical and nursing staff, and 6) use/misuse of hospital resources for those patients who may have very little benefit (Meier, 2001).

Examples of other palliative medicine programs integrated within an academic medical center include the MD Anderson Cancer Center which has a consult service, outpatient clinic and an acute inpatient palliative medicine unit (Bruera & Sweeny, 2001; Elsayem et al., 2004). Northwestern Memorial Hospital has a consultation service, an inpatient unit and a home hospice program (von Gunten, 2000).

Developing a palliative medicine program in a community setting may have its own challenges. The inpatient population has the same medical complexity has patients in academic medical centers. Being a pure consultancy service may have its disadvantages as recommendations may not be followed promptly or not at all (Cowan et al., 2002). In addition, these patients died within two weeks of the palliative medicine consultation, much shorter than those reported in an academic setting (Cowan et al., 2002). The Mount Carmel Health System started a three-hospital palliative medicine consult service in a community setting with an acute palliative care unit in each hospital (Santa-Emma et al., 2002). The Palliative Care Center of the Bluegrass incorporates strong hospice involvement in its program which includes an acute inpatient hospice unit, home hospice and home health care serving a largely rural population (Smith et al., 2004). The palliative care program at Massey Cancer Center has an inpatient palliative care unit and markets its palliative care services to its oncologists (Smith et al., 2005).

5. A Reflection on Program Development

The responsibility of caring for individuals with advanced illness can be overwhelming. Physicians, in general, lack the necessary skills needed for the complex care of these patients and often find themselves totally unprepared.

The increase in clinical fellowships in palliative medicine over the past few years is an attempt to partially correct the problem. However, it will take time before the void can be filled by adequately trained personnel.

Change is always difficult. A new venture will be scrutinized more closely and held to a higher standard than an existing service. The new program often finds itself on the defensive, either constantly proving itself or disproving misconceptions.

Program development takes time, sometimes even years to reach fruition. The patience, perseverance and energy invested to see things through can be challenging even to the most committed and the most passionate.

As the program grows and expands, requesting for additional assistance and personnel is not easy. Sometimes, the request is granted too late when existing personnel is near exhaustion and burn out.

Palliative medicine is a cognitive specialty that emphasizes decision making, medical management and psychosocial support to patients and families. It is time consuming and labor intensive. The reimbursement climate in the United States is heavily favored towards technical expertise and procedures and devalues the time and effort spent in caring for these individuals.

6. Summary

The goal of a palliative medicine program is to address the needs of individuals with advanced illness. A detailed, carefully thought of business plan written in the decision maker's language is imperative as it lays out the planning and implementation of the program in definite time intervals. Examples of models in place in several different institutions can be modified to fit the unique needs of a particular institution, whether in the academic or in the community setting. However, a comprehensive, integrated palliative medicine program will consistently provide the delivery of quality patient care and allow a structure for a financially viable program.

References

Ahmedzai SH, Walsh D. (2000). Palliative Medicine and Modern Cancer Care. *Seminars in Oncology.* 27(1):1-6.

Bruera E, Sweeney C. (2001). The development of palliative care at the University of Texas MD Anderson Cancer Center. *Support Care Cancer.* 9:330-4.

Cancer Pain Relief and Palliative Care Technical Report Series 804. Geneva, Switzerland. World Health Organization, 1990.

Cowan JD, Walsh D, Homsi J. (2002). Palliative medicine in the United States Cancer Center: a prospective study. *American Journal of Hospice and Palliative Care.* 19(4):245-50.

Cowan JD, Burns D, Palmer TW, Scott J, Feeback E. (2003). A palliative medicine program in a community setting: 12 points from the first 12 months. *American Journal of Hospice and Palliative Care.* 20(6):415-33.

Davis MP, Walsh D, LeGrand SB, Lagman R. (2002). End-of-life care: the death of palliative medicine? *Journal of Palliative Medicine.* 5(6):813-14.

Davis M, Walsh D, Nelson K, Konrad D, LeGrand S, Rybicki L. (2002). The business of palliative medicine—Part 2: The economics of acute inpatient palliative medicine. *American Journal of Hospice and Palliative Care.* 19(2):89-95.

Davis M, Walsh D, Nelson K, Konrad D, LeGrand S. (2001). The business of palliative medicine: Management metrics for an acute-care inpatient unit. *American Journal of Hospice and Palliative Care.* 18(1):26-9.

Elsayem A, Swint K, Fisch MJ, Palmer L, Reddy S, Walker P, Zhukovsky D, Knight P, Bruera E. (2004). Palliative care inpatient service in a comprehensive cancer center: clinical and financial outcomes. *Journal of Clinical Oncology.* 22(10): 2008-14.

Experton B, Ozminkowski JF, Branch LG, Li Z. (1996). A comparison by payor/provider type of the cost of dying among frail older adults. *Journal of the American Geriatric Society.* 44:1098-107.

Glare PA, Avret KA, Aggarwal G, Clark KJ, Pickstock SE, Lickiss JN. (2003). The interface between Palliative Medicine and specialists in acute-care hospitals: Boundaries, bridges and challenges. *Medical Journal of Australia.* 179 (6 suppl):529-31.

Goldstein P, Walsh D, Horvitz L. (1996). The Cleveland Clinic Foundation Harry R. Horvitz Palliative Care Center. *Supportive Care in Cancer.* 4:329-33.

Hearn J, Higginson JJ. (1998). Do specialist palliative care teams improve outcomes for cancer patients? A systematic literature review. Palliative Medicine 12(5):317-32.

Lagman R, Walsh D. (2005). Integration of palliative medicine into comprehensive cancer care. *Seminars in Oncology.* 32(2):134-8.

LeGrand S, Walsh D, Nelson K, Zhukovsky D. (2000). Development of a clinical fellowship program in palliative medicine. *Journal of Pain and Symptom Management.* 20:345-52.

Lubitz JD, Riley GF. (1993). Trends in medicine payments in the last year of life. *New England Journal of Medicine.* 328(15):1092-6.

Manfredi P, Morrison S, Goldhirsh SL, Morris EJ, Carter JM, Meier D. (2002). Palliative Care consultations: How do they impact the care of hospital patients? *Journal of Pain and Symptom Management.* 20(3):166-73.

Meier DE. Palliative care programs: what, why, and how? Physician Executive 2001, 27(6):43-7.

Meier D. (2002). United States: Overview of cancer pain and palliative care. *Journal of Pain and Symptom Management.* 24(2):265-9.

National Hospice and Palliative Care Organization: Facts and figures on hospice care in America. Arlington, VA, National Hospice and Palliative Care Organization 2003.

Nelson KA, Walsh D. (2005). The business of palliative medicine – part 3: the development of a palliative medicine program in an acute medical center. *American Journal of Hospice and Palliative Care.* 20(5):345-52.

O'Mahony S, Blank A, Zallman L, Selwyn PA. (2005). The Benefits of a Hospital-Based Inpatient Palliative Care Consultation Service: Preliminary Outcome Data. *Journal of Palliative Medicine.* 8(5):1033-9.

Pan CX, Morrison RS, Meier DE, Natale DK, Goldhirsch SL, Kralovec P, Cassel CK. (2001). How prevalent are hospital-based palliative care programs? Status report and future directions. *Journal of Palliative Medicine.* 4(3):315-24.

Santa-Emma PH, Roach R, Gill MA, Spayde P, Taylor RM. (2002). Development and implementation of an acute palliative care service. *Journal of Palliative Medicine.* 5(1):93-100.

Sheehan MK, Twaddle M. (2002). *Palliative Care Caring*. 21(10):10-1.

Smith TJ, Coyne P, Cassel B, et al. (2004). A high-volume specialist palliative care unit and team may reduce in-hospital end-of-life care costs. *Journal of Palliative Medicine*. 6(5):699-705.

Tauber C. America in transition: an aging society. Current population reports, special study series p – 23, No 128. Bureau of Census, Washington DC, US Department of Commerce, 1983.

Tropiano P, Walsh D. (2000). Organization of Services and Nursing Care: Hospice and Palliative Medicine. *Seminars in Oncology*. 27(1):7-13.

Virik K, Glare P. (2002). Profile and evaluation of a Palliative Medicine consultation service within a tertiary teaching hospital in Sydney, Australia. *Journal of Pain and Symptom Management*. 23(1):17-25.

von Gunten C. Palliative care and home hospice program Northwestern Memorial Hospital Millbank Memorial Fund 2000, 161-82.

Walsh D, Gombeski WR, Goldstein P, Hayes D, Armour M. (1994). Managing a palliative medicine oncology program: the role of a business plan. *Journal of Pain and Symptom Management*. 9(2):109-18.

Walsh D. The Harry R. Horvitz Center for Palliative Medicine, The Cleveland Clinic Foundation. Millbank Memorial Fund 2000, 51-72.

Walsh D. (2001). The Harry R. Horvitz Center for Palliative Medicine (1987-1999): Development of a novel comprehensive integrated program. *American Journal of Hospice and Palliative Care*. 18(4):239-50.

Walsh D, Gordon S. (2001). The terminally ill: dying for palliative medicine? *American Journal of Hospice and Palliative Care*. 18(3):203-5.

Walsh D. (2004). The business of palliative medicine—Part 4: Potential impact of an acute-care palliative medicine inpatient unit in a tertiary care cancer center. *American Journal of Hospice and Palliative Care*. 21(3):217-21.

Weissman D. Consultation in Palliative Medicine. *Archives of Internal Medicine*. 1997, 157(7):733-37.

www.capc.org

13

Palliative Care and Quality Management: The Core Principles of Quality Improvement and their Utility in Designing Clinical Programs for End of Life Care and Complex Case Management Models

Sarah Myers MPH* and Arthur E. Blank PhD

Over the past decade, efforts to define, build, and improve palliative care and care for complex chronic illness have been commonplace at both the micro—or organizational—and macro—or healthcare organization, payment, and regulatory policy—levels. Having grown largely out of the hospice movement, palliative care for many represents all that hospice does so well, and by extending hospice's reach offers a promise of comfortable and compassionate care earlier in the disease process than hospice is often able to.

To some, palliative care logically represents the epitome of high quality health care. Ideally palliative care is an "approach that improves the quality of life of patients and their families facing the problem associated with life-threatening illness, through the prevention and relief of suffering by means of early identification and impeccable assessment and treatment of pain and other problems, physical, psychosocial and spiritual." (World Health Organization, 2005)

The goal of this chapter is to introduce the reader to the role of simple quality improvement methods in the development and enhancement of palliative care and complex case management programs. In addition to

SARAH MYERS • Quality Improvement Consultant, Division of Health Policy & Clinical Effectiveness, Cincinnati Children's Hospital Medical Center, c/o 3333 Burnet Avenue, Cincinnati, OH 45229-3039.   ARTHUR E. BLANK • Assistant Professor, Co-Director, Division of Research, Department of Family and Social Medicine, Albert Einstein College of Medicine, 1300 Morris Park Avenue, Mazer 100, Bronx, New York 10461 and *Corresponding author: Quality Improvement Consultant, Division of Health Policy & Clinical Effectiveness, Cincinnati Children's Hospital Medical Center, c/o 3333 Burnet Avenue, Cincinnati, OH 45229-3039, Tel: 704-575-3792, e-mail: sarah.myers@cchmc.org providing background information on the need for improved quality and describing a commonly used model, we provide an example of a team seeking to infuse quality improvement into a palliative care programs, we provide the reader with suggestions for getting started with improvement, and offer some comments on how to assess the effects of these quality improvement efforts. Although quality improvement is often applied to mature programs that have discovered substantial areas for improvement in the course of care delivery, we explain that the program development phase is an ideal time to infuse quality into day-to-day activities and ensure that a program takes a proactive stance toward meeting the needs of patients and families.

1. Quality Improvement in Health Care

Over the past decade, the movement toward improvement of the quality of healthcare in the United States—with respect to outcomes, efficiency, and costs, among other things—has grown exponentially. The Institute for Healthcare Improvement (IHI, 2005), the Agency for Healthcare Research and Quality, the Institute of Medicine (IOM, 2001) and many others in the US and abroad have led the march toward a better healthcare system, pointing to inefficiency, inequity, lack of reliability, and indeed lack of safety in the very system that has made enormous strides toward reducing morbidity and mortality and eradicated many of the diseases that shortened lives as recently as 50 years ago.

IHI has been at the forefront of the movement to adapt proven improvement methods from business, engineering, and other fields to the quality problems facing the healthcare system. With Associates in Process Improvement, IHI built and disseminated the now widely-adopted Model for Improvement. (Langley et al., 1996). Using this model as a framework, they have launched numerous Breakthrough Series Collaboratives, which bring a number of healthcare provider organizations together to make breakthrough improvements in certain aspects of care, by sharing ideas for changes that can lead to improvement, networking via in-person and long-distance interaction, and reporting back to one another on the results of their efforts. (IHI, Collaborative Learning, 2005) Early Collaboratives focused on "headline-worthy" topics such as reducing Cesarean section rates and adverse drug events with later Collaboratives focusing on broader systems improvement around issues such as chronic care, palliative care, and reducing health disparities. More recently, IHI has embarked upon large-scale improvement activities aimed at creating levels of improvement that are national in scope, sustainable, and seek to achieve levels of improvement that are seemingly unattainable at first glance, including the Pursuing Perfection Project sponsored by the Robert Wood Johnson Foundation (IHI, Pursuing Perfection, 2005) and the 100,000 Lives Campaign launched in early 2005 (IHI, 2005).

1.1. IHI's Approach

The Model for Improvement developed by IHI and others is a simple, intuitive strategy for making substantial improvements in care in the context of existing staff, resources, and environmental constraints (Langley *et al.*, 1996). It is not the only quality improvement model applied successfully in a variety of health care settings and it shares many characteristics with other models and techniques, including Total Quality Management, Six Sigma strategies, and others (ASQ, 2005). We focus here on IHI's model because it has been successfully applied to the challenge of providing quality palliative care both through numerous Collaboratives beginning in the late 1990s as well as within many individual healthcare organizations (Figure 13.1).

1.2. Charting the Course

The Model for Improvement walks improvement teams through the exercise of answering three key questions, the answers of which form the roadmap for their improvement efforts. These are:

1. What are we trying to accomplish?
2. How will we know that a change is an improvement?
3. What changes can we make that will result in improvement?

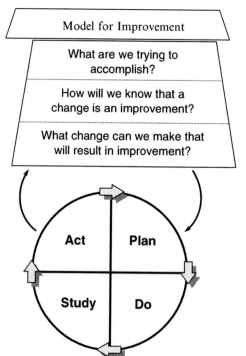

FIGURE 13.1. The model for improvement developed by associates in process improvement.

Teams confronted by these questions often wonder how such seemingly basic questions can help them frame improvement efforts. But taken together, they have, time and time again. The first question gets at the heart of the improvement project: What is our aim or our goal? What would we like to be able to say at the end of this improvement effort that we cannot say today? The second pushes a team to think about how they will track their progress toward achieving their aim: What data will they collect? Is it readily available? How often will they collect data and who will do the work? The answer to the third question leads teams to their strategies for making improvement happen—what changes will they make in processes in order to achieve improved outcomes? These strategies are often borrowed from the published literature or from other healthcare organizations, or are grassroots ideas generated by team members and others.

1.3. Try, Try, Try Again

Armed with the answers to the questions described above, improvement teams develop a simple strategy for testing the changes that they believe may lead to improvement, keeping in mind that they will likely test multiple changes over time and that the best tests start small. This part of their work hinges on the Plan-Do-Study-Act (PDSA) Cycle component of the Model for Improvement. The PDSA cycle leads a team through a series of steps aimed at determining whether their changes are leading to the outcomes that they seek to achieve and learning about the systems in which they work as they go. The components of the PDSA are as follows:

Plan: A team engaged in answering the three questions outlined above is already involved in the "Plan" part of the PDSA cycle. The team has charted a course for improvement and now must detail the steps and roles involved in their tests of change. A team that has decided to use a new pain assessment tool, for example, must now decide upon which patients they will focus, how many patients will comprise the initial test, how often the team will check in with each other to review data, and who will be responsible for implementing the various tasks involved.

Do: This is when a team gets to the real work of improvement—testing one or more their selected changes. Building on the example above, a team in the "Do" phase is on their unit or in their clinic testing the pain assessment tool on 10 cancer patients over the course of a week or on every third sickle cell patient for a month. The key is that the "doing" part is time limited and manageable within available resources. If a change is successful, a team will have plenty of opportunity to grow the size and scope of their tests and to spread it to other patient populations or parts of an organization. It is only now that many teams that are new to this model believe that they are embarked upon improvement. Indeed, many well-intentioned individuals leap into the "Do" part of the processes at from the start of an improvement effort.

Study: Once a test of change has been completed, a team that has collected data as planned will be able to step back, review the results of the test, and reflect on the lessons learned through the experience. A team testing a pain assessment tool might sit down and review pain assessment documentation in the relevant patient records to see if it is there after use of the new assessment tool. They may gather qualitative feedback from patients and staff to assess the tool's efficiency and effectiveness. By the end of this phase, they should have reached some conclusion about the success of the test and the implications for their next steps.

Act: This is where the lessons of the test are applied. A team that is satisfied that a small-scale test demonstrated that a change led to improvement might decide to expand the size of the patient population targeted. A team that saw negative effects may wish to tweak their change slightly and test it again or may wish to move on to the next change. In any case, a team moving forward to act on lessons learned in one PDSA cycle will likely find itself in the midst of more than one PDSA cycle at any given time. The team testing a pain assessment tool may make some wording and process changes and test it again, but at the same time, keeping an eye toward their overall aim of reducing pain levels, may also test the use of their organizational pain consultation service, again starting on a small scale and building up over time.

We return to measurement for a moment because though it can be the most challenging aspect of quality improvement, it is in many ways the most important—particularly during early PDSA cycles. A team testing a change will not only want to collect raw data, but also develop a simple time series chart that will help them view the data trends graphically—and ideally with annotations to assist in linking results to changes as well as external factors. Figure 13.2 shows a simple time series chart used by a team working to improve pain assessment. Note the annotations and labeling of data points. (Figure 13.2)

2. Designing Clinical Programs for End-of-Life Care and Complex Case Management Models: The Role for Quality Improvement

So far, we have described the Model for Improvement and argued that it—and other quality improvement strategies—has a role in improving palliative care. Now we turn to the why—a more detailed description of the need to infuse quality improvement not only into existing clinical situations and programs, but into new ones as well. Indeed, over the past several years, a number of organizations have taken the lead in making the business case for palliative care, most notably the Center to Advance Palliative Care at the Mount Sinai School of Medicine.i Templates of business plans, a program for visiting established palliative care programs and numerous tools for building and monitoring programs are widely available. Many organizations are seeking to

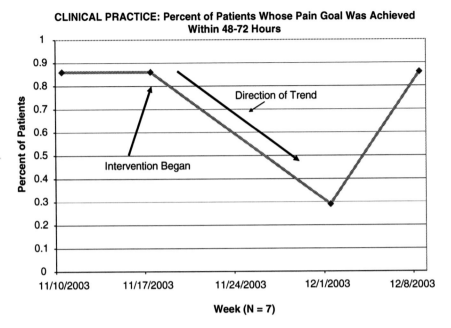

FIGURE 13.2. An example of an annotated run chart

build palliative care programs and there is strong external information and support system available to help them do so. These programs are already improving care for many patients living with serious illness and they will likely grow over the next decade. And after all, a key goal of building a program is to find a way to provide care to those who need it, and few seek to build programs that provide low quality care. So what is the role of quality improvement in new and evolving programs? Is a program not yet off the ground able to quantify what it is they would like to say about their program that they couldn't yet say today? We believe this is the ideal time to consider quality improvement—and the best way to infuse it into day-to-day activities, thereby making continuous improvement part of the culture of a program, rather than the add-on that it can often become.

As an example, a hospital contemplating the development of a palliative care program to meet the needs of seriously ill patients who do not yet qualify for hospice may initially frame this effort from a wholly program development perspective, basing decisions on market studies and business plans. We propose an alternative that infuses quality improvement from the beginning of the process—not as a replacement for solid business planning, but as a supplement. Following the core components of the Model for Improvement, the process might look like the one described below. We weave an example of an improvement team's efforts with notes about the process.

A high level planning has been assigned the task of developing a business plan for a hospital-based palliative care unit that will serve patients with cancer, chronic organ system failure, and other life-threatening diagnoses. Struggling to articulate the unique services that the program will provide—considering that the hospital already does a fine job with pain management most of the time and has experienced care managers to help many patients coordinate their care—the team asks itself a few key questions.

1. What are we trying to accomplish? The team decides to frame its aims as promises or guarantees to patients and families. What could patients and families entering the program expect as guarantees from the organization throughout their illness? The team spends a good deal of time soliciting feedback from others in the organization, as well as potential palliative care clients. The decide their initial aims are:

Aim A. Within six months of starting the program all patients in the program will state that they are confident their caregiver team has the information that they need to help them live out the end of their lives the way that they would like to.

Aim B. Within one year of starting the program, we will be able to demonstrate that 80% of patients died in their preferred setting.

Aim C. Within one year of starting the program, we will be able to demonstrate that patients never sustain levels of pain greater than 5 on a 1-10 scale for more than two hours.

Note that these aims are measurable, time-specific, and are ambitious—they are stretch aims that make clear that the team is not satisfied with the status quo. Note also that the team has avoided the common pitfall of stating changes as their aims. This is not the time to decide how they will be able to make these promises, but rather, to set the bar for performance and ensure that all stakeholders have the opportunity to contribute and buy-in to the process. Each of these aims requires some additional documentation so that it will be clear to someone outside the team exactly how the team will measure their progress. Therefore, the team selects measures to accompany each aim, answering the question:

2. How will we know that a change is an improvement? What do we need to do to track and assess our progress?

Aim A: Within six months of starting the program, all patients in the program will state within one week of admission that they are confident their caregiver team has the information that they need to help them live out the end of their lives the way that they would like to.

Measure A: The number and percent of patients who respond yes to the question: "Do you have confidence that your caregiver team has the information that they need to help you live out the end of your life the way that you would like to?"

Aim B: Within one year of starting the program, we will be able to demonstrate that 80% of patients died in their preferred setting.

Measure B: The number and percent of patients who died in the setting indicated in the medical record as their preferred place of death, as determined through medical record review or family communication.

Aim C: Within one year of starting the program, we will be able to demonstrate that patients never sustain levels of pain greater than 5 on a 1-10 scale for more than two hours.

Measure C: The number and percent of patients with documented pain levels that exceed 5 on a 1-10 scale on initial and 2-hour post-intervention pain assessment.

It is one thing to solidify measures that fit a team's aims and accurately capture the level of improvement achieved. It is another to actually implement a measurement plan. Where to find the data? Who to collect the data? How often? These are vital questions that can lead to substantial confusion and anxiety within an improvement team. Clearly, data describing the selected measures would be too cumbersome to collect for all patients, all the time. Depending on the size of the patient population, improvement teams selected to shepherd progress toward each of the aims will want to select a reasonable sample size and data collection and reporting schedule, as illustrated in the continuation of our example:

The team assigned to Aim C, related to pain levels, realizes that a palliative care program serving up to 50 patients at any given time will not be able to track daily— or more frequent—pain scores for every patient, every day. Such a data collection effort could be someone's full time job. Therefore, the team decides that once a week, a nursing assistant will be assigned to review at least 10 current patients' charts, noting on a simple data collection log all instances in the past week that patients' documented pain levels exceeded 5 on a 1-10 scale on both initial and 2-hour post-intervention pain assessment. Over time, if the nurse finds that the review is not too cumbersome, she may add more charts to her weekly review.

With this challenge solved, the team turns to determining the best way to collate the collected data and put it into a format from which they can learn about the effectiveness of their efforts.

The teams decides that once a month, the nursing assistant who conducts the chart reviews will give the data abstraction logs to the nurse manager. The nurse manager will enter the data into a simple spreadsheet and from that build a time series chart that the team can use for data analysis and learning.

With a data collection and management strategy in mind, the team can proceed with the real work of improvement—deciding how they are going to get there. This is where they answer the third question.

3. What changes can we make that will result in improvement? The team realizes that there are many steps needed to achieve their aim related to patients' pain levels. For one thing, they want to ensure that pain is indeed being assessed through a standardized process. After gathering information about current hospital pain assessment strategies and the positive and negative aspects of the various approaches, the team selects a process that they believe is worth testing to start. They also know from experience that pain levels are recorded in the medical record. The team decides that they will test the use of a pain assessment log for inclusion in the front of the record. Finally, the team knows that assessment does not guarantee improvement and they select a pain response protocol that has been used successfully by another medical center.

As described earlier in this chapter, changes are tested via a series of PDSA cycles, with teams learning from these tests and building upon them as they continue to work toward achieving their aims.

3. Getting Started

3.1. Where to Aim

Some readers of this text will be working in the context of a formal palliative care program; many others will not. In either case, although palliative care is an area that is ripe for improvement, it can be hard getting started with developing aims. It can be helpful to think about shortcomings that one regularly sees in the care of very ill patients in one or more of the following domains (Lynn *et al.*, 2000).

Advance care planning: Are patients that wish to die at home dying in the hospital? Are patients religious and other preferences being ignored or not solicited at all? Are patients given unrealistic expectations about their future when they actually have a rather predictable disease course?

Pain and other symptom management: Are patients waiting too long for effective pain management between outpatient visits? Are chronic obstructive pulmonary disease patients living with crippling dyspnea? Are patients with dementia assumed to be pain free because finding a pain assessment scale to use with them is challenging?

Continuity and coordination of care: Are families complaining about the fact that they give the same information to multiple providers in the same day? Are nursing home patients being needlessly transferred to the hospital in the last days of life? Are elderly patients with complex medical needs experiencing medication errors due the complexity of their management?

Patient and family education and support: Are family complaints too common to notice? Are patients who are capable of self-care missing the opportunity due to lack of educational resources? Are families of seriously ill children being left out of important medical decisions?

Beginning with this short set of questions can help an individual—or an improvement team—begin to frame their aims. While not downplaying the need for some process measures, the key is to stay focused on outcomes. It is much more satisfying to demonstrate an improvement in patients' symptom burden or a families' satisfaction with the care their loved one received before death than to report on a committee's efforts do develop a new policy or form, or even on the development of a new, state-of-the-art program.

3.2. Building an Improvement Team

We emphasized early in this chapter that the Model for Improvement encouraging small scale tests of change, at least at the beginning of an improvement project. A benefit of this characteristic is that just one person can conceivably come up with an aim, test of series of changes, and learn from the resulting data. However, most areas in need of improvement in healthcare can benefit from—and indeed require—the involvement of several people who are close to the process in need of improvement. The Model for Improvement is best implemented when there are a few key roles filled within a team:

Team leader: This is the person who convenes the team, seeks out other appropriate participants and makes sure that the work is implemented.

Technical Expert: This is usually a clinician with strong skills in the area of focus. For example, within a team working on pain issues, this is often a physician with extensive pain management experience and expertise.

System leader: This is a person who can serve as a liaison with organizational leadership, ensuring that the teams aims are in line with organizational goals and who can help troubleshoot around resource and constraints. This may be a clinical division manager, a physician leader, or other individual who has access to the upper levels of an organization.

Beyond these core roles, the team should be populated by individuals with "ownership" of the issue being addressed. A team working on pain may not include a chaplain, whereas a team working on advance care planning likely will. A team working on transfers and continuity in a nursing home will want to included care managers, admissions representatives, the other relevant clinical staff, and perhaps even a family representative.

The team described in our example set out to build a palliative care program, but by infusing good quality improvement principles, they avoid building a program that looked good on paper but were unable to document quality outcomes that really matter to clinicians, patients and families—which is key to both good care and often to access to additional resources. By building a quality improvement infrastructure into the core fabric of the program, the team is more likely to find itself in the situation of reporting to a Board, potential patients and their families, and their current and potential staff that their program was designed around the needs of patients and families, rather than that they are figuring out the needs of patients and families by trial and error as they go along. Of course any team encounters unanticipated problems, and many quality improvement initiatives are less successful than they are educational. As new or persistent quality problems emerge, new quality improvement projects can be implemented.

3.3. Pitfalls to Avoid

There are a number of pitfalls to avoid in the course of these projects. Getting underway with improvement activities anchored by weak, non-specific aims is the best way to launch an unsuccessful effort. Aims that are not measurable and time specific lack the clarity needed to demonstrate to the team—and others—that the team is holding itself accountable to a common—and important—goal. Stating aim in general terms, such as "We will improve advance care planning for cancer patients," makes clear that a team wants to improve something, but does not set a timeline or threshold for the team to rally around. The aim should also be in line with organizational priorities. For example, an organization that does not include symptom management within its overall strategic plan or organizational goals may not be the most hospitable place for a team addressing these issues.

3.4. Measures

Many improvement teams hesitate to test changes that sound too simple, or for which there is little solid evidence of their ability to improve care. For example, teams working to improve palliative care have tested changes such as including an attending physician's beeper number on hospice patients' medical records in order to more easily reach him or her in case of emergency. This seems quite simple at first glance, but no one thought of it until they critically examined the current system that led to long waits for adequate pain management. If an idea sounds like it could work in a particular setting, it is usually worth a try. Testing changes that are limited in scope with a small group of patients allows an improvement team to try and "fail" with few negative consequences. It is much easier to earn the leeway to test another change when the first has not caused substantial staff distraction from day-to-day duties, wasted resources, or patients and families that are worse off than they were before.

Selecting and defining measures for a quality improvement effort raise numerous challenges to the team and one should be briefly mentioned: the validity of the measures used. To the extent possible it is preferable to use validated measures–both outcome and process measures. However, many published measures require resources, staff and time, not always available to QI teams. Consequently, compromises will have to be made or new measures devised that are more directly responsive to the improvement strategy put in place. The result is that some measures will have an intuitive meaning for the team and the institution, face validity if you will, but lack the rigor of traditional research measures. Teams need to be aware of this tradeoff. It should be noted, however, that using validated measures to address a question the team is not interested in answering is also a measurement error.

4. Conclusion

The goal of this chapter was to introduce the reader to the role of simple quality improvement methods in the development of palliative care programs, focusing on the Institute for Healthcare Improvement's Model for Improvement. We provided an example of a team seeking to build such a program and provided suggestions for getting started with improvement. Palliative care is the purview of providers from a number of settings, specialties, and educational backgrounds; the methods we have described here can be readily applied to other areas of practice. Regulatory, consumer, and other demands will continue to create ample opportunities for clinicians and allied health providers to get involved as leaders of quality improvement initiatives.

As these QI initiative grow, it is essential to raise a critical question-what is the evidence that these QI strategies lead to improved outcomes? There is no evidence yet in palliative care. If we look at more established collaboratives, i.e., collaboratives working with chronic illnesses where there is an accepted and valid outcome measure (e.g., A1c levels in diabetes), the evidence is inconclusive (Ferlie and Shortell, 2001; Mittman, 2004; Ovretveit et al., 2002; Landon et al., 2004; Cretin et al., 2004; Baier et al., 2004). Consequently, institutionally specific, pragmatic QI efforts need to be supplemented by rigorous, ethically responsible, well designed and conducted research projects that test a critical presumption of QI efforts that have migrated to health care – do rapid cycle testing, and routine data collection on well established outcome measures lead to improved outcomes?. While process change may lead directly to the desired outcomes in stable, relatively static systems, the route may be decidedly less direct in complex systems such as health care organizations that are both dynamic and reactive to external and internal pressures.

References

American Society for Quality. About Quality. Available online: http://www.asq.org/portal/ Accessed March 1, 2005.

Baier RR, Giffrd DR, Patry G, Banks SM, ROchon T, SeSilva D, Teno JN, (2004) Ameliorating Pain in Nursing Homes: A Collaborative Quality Improvement Project, *Journal of the American Geriatrics Society.* 52:1988-1995.

Cretin S, Shortell SM, Keeler EB, (2004), An Evaluation of Collaborative Interventions to Improve Chronic Illness Care: Framework and Study Design, *Evaluation Review.* 28(1):28-51.

Ferlie EB, Shortell SM, 2001, Improving the Quality of Health Care in the United Kingdom and the United States: A Framework for Change, *The Milbank Quarterly.* 79(2):281-314.

Institute for Healthcare Improvement. 2005. Institute for Healthcare Improvement 2005 Progress Report. Available online: www.ihi.org. Accessed March 1, 2005.

Institute of Medicine. Crossing the Quality Chasm: A New Health System for the 21st Century. Washington, DC: National Academy Pr; 2001.

Institute for Healthcare Improvement. Collaborative Learning. Available online: http://ihi.org/IHI/Programs/CollaborativeLearning/. Accessed March 1, 2005.

Institute for Healthcare Improvement. Pursuing Perfection: Raising the Bar for Health Care Performance. Available online: http://ihi.org/IHI/Programs/PursuingPerfection/. Accessed March 1, 2005.

Institute for Healthcare Improvement. 100k Lives Campaign. Available online: http://ihi.org/IHI/Programs/Campaign/. Accessed March 1, 2005.

Landon BE, Wilson IR, McInnes K, Landrum MB, Hirschorn L, Mardsen PV, Gustafson D, Cleary P, (2004) Effects of a Quality Improvement Collaborative on the Outcome of Care of Patients with HIV infection: The EQHIV study, *Annals of Internal Medicine.* 140(11):888-896.

Langley GL, Nolan KM, Nolan TW, Norman CL, Provost LP. 1996. The Improvement Guide. San Francisco, California, USA: Jossey-Bass Publishers.

Lynn J, Schuster JL, Kabcenell A. Improving Care for the End of Life: A Sourcebook for Health Care Managers and Clinicians. New York: Oxford Univ Pr; 2000.

Mittman BS, (2004) Creating the Evidence Base for Quality Improvement Collaboratives, *Annals of Internal Mediciine.* 140(11):897-901.

Ovretveit J, Bate P, Clearly P, Cretin S, Gustafson D, McInnes K, McLeod H, Molfenter T, Pisek P, Robert G, Shortell S, Wilson T, (2002) Quality collaboratives: lessons from research, *Qual Saf Health Care.* 11:345-351.

World Health Organization. WHO Definition of Palliative Care. Available online: http://www.who.int/cancer/palliative/definition/en/. Accessed: January 27, 2005.

14
Ethics and the Delivery of Palliative Care

Linda Faber-Post JD BSN MA

1. The Intersection of Ethics and Palliation

Bioethics is about decisions in health care—how they are made, by whom and based on what considerations. In the clinical, organizational and policy settings, hard choices require the appreciation of profound consequences and the sensitive balancing of rights, principles and interests. Core ethical principles that provide an analytic framework for decision making and give rise to professional obligations include respecting autonomy (supporting and facilitating the capable patient's exercise of self-determination); beneficence (promoting the patient's best interest and well-being, and protecting the patient from harm); nonmaleficence (avoiding actions likely to cause the patient harm); and distributive justice (allocating fairly the benefits and burdens related to health care delivery) (Beauchamp and Childress, 2001). Among the most challenging decisions are those related to the goals of care, the limits of medicine, the boundaries of hope, and the imperatives of compassion. The integrity with which these decisions are made and implemented is the mutual concern of bioethics and palliative care.

While providing comfort, especially at the end of life, has been part of the traditional responsibilities of the caring professions, the advent of biotechnology shifted the focus to the cure of disease and disability. Palliative care as a discipline has successfully reintroduced the notion that relieving pain and suffering is central to the complete and authentic practice of medicine (Bretscher and Creagan, 1997). Its defining philosophy is the conviction that cure and comfort are consistent objectives that may assume greater or lesser prominence, depending on the patient's condition, prognosis and values. The issues addressed by both palliative care and bioethics—dignity, suffering, comfort, death, relationships, self-identity, vulnerability, truth, trust, hope—are

---

LINDA FABER-POST • Bioethicist and Clinical Ethics Consultant.

among the most profound because they help to define the human condition. Regardless of ethnicity, gender, age, socioeconomic or educational status, people grapple with questions about the meaning and quality of their existence, especially at life's most pivotal moments. Helping patients, families and professionals to adjust their goals and make decisions in ways that have clinical and ethical validity is the contribution of bioethics (Post *et al.*, 2006; Post and Dubler, 1997).

1.1. The Moral Imperative to Relieve Pain and Suffering

As discussed at greater length elsewhere (Post *et al.*, 1996), the relief of pain is more than a professional obligation. It has traditionally been considered a moral imperative for those who minister to the sick. Even when cure has not been possible, the mandate to comfort has defined the caregiver role. Palliation also illustrates the tension between two fundamental ethical principles, autonomy and beneficence. The dual obligation of clinicians is to respect and promote their patients' autonomy *and* to protect and enhance their well-being. The preoccupation of Western (largely Anglo-American) cultures with self-determination, however, has elevated the notion of autonomy to a position of primacy, reflected in the centrality of informed consent in the clinical setting. Under this doctrine, capable, knowledgeable and voluntary consent is required for legally and ethically valid authorization of most diagnostic and therapeutic interventions.

Yet, the requirement of informed consent is conspicuously absent from the relief of pain because, in the palliative setting, the principle of beneficence is elevated even over autonomy. This imperative is so strong that it gives rise to the presumption that, absent explicit objection, those in pain would want their discomfort relieved. Thus, the capable patient's clearly articulated decision to refuse analgesia must be honored, but the vulnerable incapacitated patient must not be deprived of pain relief because of an inability to provide consent. Relieving pain is central to the very notion of healing and, for that reason alone, it requires no additional justifications.

1.2. The Imperative Unmet

Despite the well-established moral imperative to relieve pain, however, patients both with and without capacity routinely receive inadequate palliation throughout the therapeutic continuum, even at the end of life (Desbiens *et al.*, 1996). Studies have demonstrated that similar pain complaints from patients with similar injuries were met with different analgesic responses associated with ethnicity (Todd *et al.*, 1993), age and gender stereotyping (Calderone, 1990), and disparities between physician and patient assessment of pain (Todd *et al.*, 1994). The several reasons for insufficient pain management implicate personal and cultural values related to character and dependence; perceptions about age, gender, race and ethnicity and their influence on how pain is experienced and expressed; clinician misinformation about pain, analgesic agents and addiction; and physician concerns about opioid prescription and legal liability (Alpers, 1998; Post *et al.*, 1996).

Numerous studies have shown that inadequate professional education about analgesia, misconceptions about opioids and addiction, fears about regulatory and legal liability inhibit clinicians from adequately responding to pain. Physicians' concerns about giving opioids that depress respiration while relieving pain include their ethical obligations of nonmaleficence, expressed in the maxim "first, do no harm," and their fears of legal liability (Foley, 1995; SUPPORT Principal Investigators, 1995; Zenz, 1991). Considerable pharmacologic knowledge and clinical skill are required to achieve adequate analgesia, and the increasing involvement of palliative care specialists provides an invaluable resource.

A critical distinction supporting adequate palliation at the end of life is the doctrine of double effect, which holds that a single act having two foreseen effects, one good and one bad, is not morally or legally prohibited *if the harmful effect is not intended.* The doctrine recognizes that, while the administration of sufficient opioids to manage pain at the end of life risks depressing respirations enough to hasten death, the clinical and ethical mandate to relieve suffering is paramount.

Using the rationale of the doctrine of double effect, the palliative intervention is both approved and protected. Indeed, no less a legal authority than the U.S. Supreme Court has explicitly distinguished palliation, forgoing unwanted medical treatment, and assisted suicide, and affirmed the validity of the doctrine of double effect. In the landmark 1997 cases, *Washington v. Glucksberg* and *Vacco v. Quill*, the Court ruled that, while there is no constitutionally protected right to physician assistance in committing suicide, there is a protected liberty interest in adequate pain relief at the end of life. Helping physicians appreciate this distinction so that they can comfortably provide adequate palliation is often part of ethics intervention.

1.3. Racial and Ethnic Disparities in Palliative Care

The moral imperative to relieve pain is also inhibited by societal barriers to palliative care, an unacceptable situation that implicates the ethical principle of distributive justice. Particularly disturbing are repeated reports of racial and ethnic disparities in health care, including diagnostic, curative, life-sustaining and palliative interventions (Wolf, 2004; Epstein and Ayania, 2001; Phillips *et al.*, 1996). Studies have revealed that in the emergency setting (Todd *et al.*, 2000), the post-operative setting (Ng *et al.*, 1996), and the outpatient setting (Cleeland *et al.*, 1994, 1997), minority patients were more likely to receive inadequate analgesia than nonminority patients. A 2001 study of pharmacies in all five New York City boroughs revealed that, while 72% of pharmacies in predominantly white neighborhoods stocked opioids sufficient to treat severe pain, only 25% of pharmacies in predominantly nonwhite neighborhoods had these drugs available (Morrison *et al.*, 2000).

These reports are of special concern because of what they reveal about both effect and cause. The health consequences of disparate care are reflected in the reported underuse among non white patients of diagnostic and therapeutic interventions projected to improve clinical outcomes. Moreover, these disparities have remained relatively unchanged for decades in the United States, as has the average life expectancy of blacks, which is six years shorter than that of whites (Epstein and Ayaian, 2001; Freeman and Payne, 2000). According to one estimate, compared to the vast sums dedicated to improving medical technology in an effort to save lives, five times as many deaths could be averted if the disparities in health care were corrected (Woolf, 2004).

Racial disparities in medical services suggest possible discrimination or bias, either deliberate or unintentional, by health care providers, including clinicians and institutions. It is also argued that the causes of the inequities implicate health care systems rather than just individual providers, and will need to be addressed systemically (Epstein and Ayaian, 2001; Freeman and Payne, 2000). Although the disparities in health care tend to fall along racial and ethnic lines, commentators caution against viewing the problem as stemming only from patients' cultural values and provider discrimination. Rather, it has been suggested that the overarching problems are the socioeconomic conditions of marginalized populations and the societal priorities that do not have as a goal a "common standard of wellness." What is lacking, then, may not be the national resources to create a just health care system, but the national resolve (Woolf, 2004).

1.4. The Business of Palliative Care

Traditionally, ethical scrutiny and analysis have focused on the issues in health care that arise in the clinical, research and social policy settings. Matters of concern have included treatment decision making, the physician-patient relationship, care at the beginning and end of life, research with human subjects, and the just allocation of health care resources. Increasingly, however, the scope of attention is expanding to encompass organizational issues. This relatively new perspective is premised on the notion that health care organizations, as well as individual clinicians, are moral agents with obligations to the people who depend on them. Responding to the transformation of health care from a physician-patient interaction to a corporate management dynamic, organizational ethics concerns itself with how the business of medicine affects the delivery of care. In this view, health care organizations are held morally accountable for their actions as revealed in their policies and decisions (Blustein *et al.*, 2004; Blustein *et al.*, 2002).

The analytic framework of organizational ethics has particular relevance to the objectives and functioning of palliative care. As the specialty secures its place in the health care landscape, it is encountering the challenges of defining its clinical identity and goals, distinguishing its role as a resource and provider of quality care, and ensuring its fiscal viability. For example, considerable attention has been directed to the question of whether the focus should be on care at the end of life or move more "upstream" to encourage earlier and broader involvement of palliative specialists in the therapeutic continuum. Some commentators argue that the "end-of-life" label restricts and even stigmatizes palliative care, discouraging physician referral and patient involvement in the same way as the "hospice" designation. They reason that palliation encompasses preventive and chronic, as well as terminal, care, co-managing a wide variety of illnesses not typically associated with death and dying (Davis *et al.*, 2002). The counter argument is that trying to adapt the symptom management skills of palliative care to the entire acute and chronic continuum dilutes the expertise that the specialty can bring to the care of the dying (Arnold, 2002).

The tension between the obligations to provide high quality care and control costs, inherent in managed care, is especially important in the provision of palliative care. Studies have shown that, during the last year of life, the majority of medical costs are incurred during the final 30-60 days. Yet, the implications of these expenditures are nothing less than life and death. Because decisions about end-of-life care are costly in terms of both finances and clinical outcome, initiatives have focused on developing palliative care systems that manage patients' chronic and terminal care needs while appropriately allocating limited resources. The challenge, requiring both clinical and ethical vigilance, is to promote fiscal responsibility without limiting patient choice or sacrificing quality of care (Smith *et al.*, 2003; Brumley, 2002; Walsh *et al.*, 1994).

2. Clinical Ethics Collaboration in Palliative Care

While symptom management should be an integral part of the entire therapeutic continuum, intensive focus on palliation is typically an indication that the end of life is approaching. The issues that are raised and the decisions they require, which are discussed in the following sections, are some of the most difficult encountered in the clinical setting. Usually these decisions are made by the patient or, more often, the patient's family and the care team.

Sometimes, however, the complex nature of the decisions and their profound consequences create confusion or disagreement, usually involving the patient's decisional capacity, the obligation of the care professionals to promote the patient's interests, and differences in how the goals and plan of care are perceived. When these clinical conflicts occur, a bioethics consultation can be especially helpful in gathering the key parties and ensuring that they have the same information, clarifying the issues, providing a forum for deliberation, helping to define the goals of care and the therapeutic options, identifying the relevant ethical principles, and supporting the parties in resolving the conflict in ways that are mutually acceptable.

Institutions differ in how clinical ethics consultations are requested, conducted and documented. In some facilities, the request must come through the attending physician, while in others it may come from anyone involved in the patient's care, including house staff, nurses, social workers, patient services representatives, risk managers or hospital counsel, the patient or family. The consultation, conducted by a trained ethicist or an ad hoc group of the institution's ethics committee, may involve the patient, family and the care team and is usually documented in the progress notes or as a formal clinical consultation note (Back and Arnold, 2005; Dubler and Liebman, 2004; Post, 2003).

3. Ethical Issues in the Clinical Palliative Care Setting

3.1. Making Decisions at the End-of-Life

An ethics analysis considers the goals and plan of care in light of the patient's condition and prognosis, the benefits, burdens and risks of the treatment options, and what is known of the patient's wishes. As a rule, the course of care is determined by the capable patient, based on personal values and an understanding of the available choices. Preferably, these decisions are guided and supported by the professionals caring for the patient, drawing on their clinical judgment and knowledge of the patient's wishes. This ideal, however, should be tempered by the caution that the concepts and principles of American bioethics reflect mainly Western values and that the notion of autonomy is essentially a product of Western preoccupation with individuality and self-reliance (Jecker et al., 1995; Pellegrino, 1993). Pellegrino has argued that viewing health care decision making only through the lens of autonomy risks preventing care providers from recognizing that some patients may not want to make health care decisions and that beneficence and respect include adapting to multicultural considerations and not imposing an unwanted burden of autonomous decision making (Pellegrino, 1992).

Decision making in the face of terminal illness requires a heightened level of commitment and courage on the part of both the capable patient and the caregivers. The optimism that pervades collaborative planning for care that is expected to cure or improve the patient's condition is often replaced with sadness, fear, denial and anger. Rather than looking forward to a return to health and fitness, the patient is asked to anticipate a decline in vitality and function.

The more common and difficult scenario in palliative care, however, concerns decision making by others for patients without capacity, usually at the end of life. These situations require surrogates, typically family members, to draw on what they know of the patient's values and preferences, envisioning what that person would want in the current circumstances. Sometimes, prospective instructions or prior conversations provide clear guidance about what the patient would choose if able to do so.

Responding to the need for decision making on behalf of incapacitated patients, two approaches have developed: advance directives and surrogate decision making. Advance directives are legal mechanisms that permit capable persons to articulate their preferences about care so that, when capacity is lost, their wishes can be communicated and implemented. They were conceived during the 1970s in response to growing concerns that patients without the ability to make care decisions risked being subjected to unwanted interventions, especially at the end of life.

Living wills are written lists of instructions about interventions that patients do or do not want under specified circumstances, usually at the end of life. These directives are limited by their static nature and the requirement that persons executing them anticipate their possible future medical conditions and what they will want under those circumstances. In contrast, health care proxy appointments (also known as durable powers of attorney for health care), permit the capable person to legally appoint another individual (a health care agent) who assumes the authority to make health care decisions on behalf of the patient if and when capacity is lost. This preferred type of advance directive provides the flexibility to enable the agent to interact with the care team and respond to unanticipated and changing clinical conditions (Post, 2005).

The early promise of advance directives has been only partially realized and considerable research has revealed some of the factors that either impede or promote their utility. Although the Patient Self-Determination Act (PSDA) requires that all care-providing institutions receiving federal funding provide new patients with information about advance directives, only 15-25% of the United States adult population has either a living will or a health care proxy (Gillick, 2004; Wissow *et al.*, 2004). It is worth noting, however, that initiatives, such as a concerted advance directive education program (Hammes and Rooney, 1998) and efforts targeting physician education and behavior (Wissow *et al.*, 2004), have been shown to increase advance directive execution and implementation.

Studies have shown that physicians are often unaware of their patients' advance directives; health care agents make decisions that do not always reflect patient wishes; and even physician knowledge of patient preferences does not always affect treatment decisions (Lo and Steinbrook, 2004; Prendergast, 2001; SUPPORT investigators, 1995; Morrison *et al.*, 1995). Rather than deliberate provider disregard, however, the failure of advance directives to accurately influence care decisions reflects the unavailability of previously executed directives when patients are admitted to acute care hospitals; serious patient misconceptions about the interventions they are requesting or refusing; physician inability to predict patient treatment preferences, uncertainty about the applicability of the directives' provisions, and lack of consensus about how to interpret their intent. These studies reveal the need for earlier, more frequent and better communication between patients and physicians, focusing on the goals of care rather than specific interventions. Ideally, advance care planning should be a *process* of mutual patient-physician education rather than simply a legal ratification of a poorly understood decision (Teno *et al.*, 1998; Fischer *et al.*, 1998; Loewy, 1998; Gross, 1998; Morrison *et al.*, 1998).

More often, however, the explicit authorization and guidance of an advance directive is lacking and treatment decisions require inferences based on recalled comments or behaviors. Unfortunately, conversations about these decisions typically take place in the least opportune circumstances—in the acute care setting at the time of a sentinel event when the unresponsive patient is in multi-organ system failure, the family is under enormous stress, and professionals seek guidance in care planning. Not infrequently, families anticipating aggressive treatment to produce clinical improvement will withhold information about patient wishes regarding life-sustaining interventions, particularly ventilatory support. This information may be shared only after it is clear that the patient will almost certainly not return to baseline (O'Mahony et al., 2003).

Relevant information can often be elicited by care givers willing to invest the time and effort in helping surrogates search their memories. "Did Mama ever talk about her brother's dying?" "What care decisions did your sister make for her husband when he was so ill?" "Did your father ever know anyone who was on dialysis or a breathing machine?" "What did your aunt find most frightening or distressing about being sick?" This arduous and stressful process can be facilitated if surrogates are reassured that their contribution is to provide information about the patient's values and wishes, not to assume sole responsibility for making critical decisions, and that all clinically indicated measures likely to benefit the patient will be pursued.

3.2. Sharing the Burden of Making Difficult Decisions

The prevailing emphasis on promoting the exercise of autonomy and respecting patient choice risks diminishing the importance of the clinician role in care planning. Treatment decisions require a grasp of often complex medical data, as well as insight into the patients personal goals and values. Decisions about end-of-life care, in particular, can be emotionally wrenching. Both professionalism and compassion dictate that the burden of making them be shared by those responsible for the care Patients and families depend on professional guidance in making hard decisions and depriving them of clinical judgment, advice and support can be seen as a form of abandonment. Palliative care clinicians have both the opportunity and the obligation to provide patients and families with information, guidance and support, including candor and clarity about medical uncertainty and the limits of what medicine can accomplish.

Choices should not be presented as value neutral when one approach is clearly preferable. Rather, the benefits, burdens, risks and alternatives should be clearly outlined, along with the physician's clear recommendation and rationale. Also, states differ in their standards for withholding or withdrawing life-sustaining treatments; some accord families considerable decision-making authority, while others require clear and convincing evidence of the patient's wishes. Although legal constraints may shape the discussion, they cannot justify physician abdication of the responsibility to define its realistic parameters. Guiding patient or family decisions should not be confused with paternalism, which demeans the capable adult and constricts the exercise of self-determination. In contrast, offering guidance and support enhances the ability to act in ways that promote dignity and well-being.

Physicians caring for critically ill patients are often faced with patient or family instructions to "do everything" or requests for specific interventions judged to be therapeutically ineffective or otherwise inappropriate. These discussions often invoke the notion of medical futility to explain why proposed treatments are not clinically indicated. Despite considerable effort, an agreed-upon determination of futility remains elusive. Its narrowest and most useful definition describes the *physiologic impossibility* of an intervention achieving its therapeutic objective. In that strict sense, physicians are excused from burdening patients with treatment that will be clinically ineffective (Youngner, 1988).

Far more often, however, interventions are labeled futile when they are expected to produce a clinical effect that falls below a specified standard, which may include producing a particular physiologic effect, extending life, or enhancing comfort and function. Differing values and expectations of the patient, family and care team may prevent consensus on the definition of success, contributing to confusion and conflict about the meaning of futility (Luce, 1995).

In addition to definitional inconsistency, the notion of futility suffers from prognostic fallibility. The technical difficulty in precisely predicting clinical outcomes is compounded by the stress physicians associate with patient, family and colleague expectations of certainty, concerns about potential negative reactions to prognostic errors, and discomfort with determining and communicating unfavorable prognoses. These problems are magnified in palliative care where concepts, such as "terminally ill" and "dying," may lack precision (Christakis and Iwashyna, 1998; Arnold, 2002). Even computer-based models, useful in estimating survival in patient populations, have limited utility in predicting individual patient outcomes (Lemeshow *et al.*, 2004).

Mindful of their conflicting obligations to provide only beneficial treatments, avoid interventions that risk significant harm, not raise unrealistic expectations, and deliver cost-effective care, physicians may label questionably effective interventions "futile" as a way of withholding them in specific instances. Futility can also function as the trump card to discourage families from insisting on treatment that care providers consider inappropriate.

Some commentators argue that physicians should not be the arbiters of which requested interventions should or should not be provided. The reasoning is that, because of medical prognostic uncertainty, lack of professional consensus on notions of futility, concern about cost of care and resource constraints, and their own personal values, physicians are not well-suited to determine the reasonableness of most treatment requests. Rather, it is suggested that defining beneficence and best interest should be the responsibility of the patient and family, for whom the desired interventions have the most significance (Sprung *et al.*, 1995).

While notions of quality of life, dignity and self-determination are certainly subjective and are most authentically interpreted by the patients or those who know them best, assuming that all treatment requests, however clinically counterproductive, should be honored seems an abdication of physician responsibility. Decisions to forgo treatments unlikely to benefit individual patients should not be confused with resource rationing to benefit society, questions that raise issues of distributive justice rather than clinical effectiveness and should not be addressed at the bedside. Providing guidance in choosing the most therapeutically effective course for each patient has traditionally been and remains central to the physician-patient interaction.

Requests to "do everything" should be seen as an important signal that the parties to the interaction may not share the same understanding of the patient's condition and prognosis, the goals of care, the available treatment options, and the expected outcomes of the requested interventions. Family members often feel an obligation as good advocates to ensure that their loved ones are not neglected and that no treatment is left untried. Especially when they are uncertain what to anticipate or how much confidence to place in the care team, they may request all available therapies in the hope that one of them will be effective.

Like treatment refusals, insistence on inappropriate treatment should trigger further discussion and clarification. Among the first things to determine are what "everything" means to those making the request and what the interventions in question are expected to accomplish. Specific requests should be considered in light of their clinical indication and the likelihood that they will advance the care plan. Discussion should focus on clarifying the goals of care, the likely effectiveness of the proposed treatments in achieving those goals, and the obligation to prevent suffering without benefit.

3.3. Protecting Patients from Treatment

Among the most difficult decisions in palliative care are those related to forgoing treatment at the end of life. Decisions about continuing or terminating life-sustaining interventions, thereby deferring or permitting death, are painful and often paralyzing for those who are asked to act on behalf of their loved ones. Left to make these choices alone, the family or other surrogate is likely to feel solely responsible for the outcome. Here, too, clinicians have an obligation to shoulder part of the burden of decision making.

How decisions about forgoing treatment are handled depends greatly on how they are framed. Withholding or withdrawing specific interventions can be seen as *depriving* the patient of needed therapy, decreasing care, or simply giving up. Patients and families, afraid of being abandoned, are understandably resistant to the notion of limiting care.

An alternative approach, consistent with the palliative philosophy, focuses on the ethical mandate to relieve suffering and prevent harm by *protecting* the patient from the burden of unnecessary, ineffective interventions. The emphasis is on identifying and providing only treatment that will benefit the patient, eliminating the selected interventions that fail to meet that standard. When continued treatment will only prolong the dying process or increase suffering without corresponding benefit, it is appropriate to help the patient's loved ones give themselves permission to make hard choices that will be in his best interest. Toward this end, the notion of family as protector at the end of life can be a powerful and comforting one that should be reinforced.

3.4. Palliative Care: Giving Up or Giving Permission

While the shift in goals from cure to comfort is a process rather than a sudden decision, there comes a time when the care team, family and, often, the patient should acknowledge that palliation is now the focus of care. Recognizing and accepting this reality is unlike other care decisions because of the profound implications for everything that follows. For many people, including patients, families and physicians, reliance on palliative care is accompanied by a sense of loss and defeat (Arnold, 2002). The expectation of cure, sometimes even the hope for improvement, must be relinquished. The belief in the power of medicine is exchanged for frustration and lingering doubts about whether all possible options have been explored. The common but unfortunate distinction between "aggressive" and "comfort" care reinforces the notion that palliation represents a lesser level of attention and commitment while waiting for death. The unintended but clear message is, "We have given up and you should too."

A common response to the suggestion that palliative care be consulted is, "Are things really that hopeless?" or "He'll lose all hope." While patient and family resistance to a palliative care plan is often explained as denial of impending death or concern that less attentive care will be provided, the more profound fear appears to be the relinquishing of hope.

The perception can and should be reframed. Rather than abandoning hope, the move to palliative care can be seen as liberating the patient, family and care team from increasingly counterproductive efforts to reverse the inexorably deteriorating clinical course. The clear message should be that hope need not be the price of palliation, but an integral part of it. With the investment of time and skill, those who care for and about the patient can give themselves permission to focus on an aggressive care plan that will enhance the quality of the life that remains. Indeed, the therapeutic options can be expanded. Precisely because palliation remains on the care continuum after cure is no longer the goal, it may encompass particular comfort measures posing risks to life, including higher doses of more potent medication, which might not have been acceptable when cure was still the goal of care. Rather than "Death is approaching and it must be resisted as long as possible," the message becomes "Life is continuing and its quality must be enhanced as much as possible."

4. Conclusion

Throughout the therapeutic continuum, from the diagnosis of illness to the moment of death, the concerns and goals of care giving include maximizing the benefits and minimizing the burdens of treatment, palliating suffering and empowering patients and families to make principled and value-based decisions, enhance the quality of their lives, and retain a measure of hope in the future. Given their shared vision of and commitment to patient well-being, the continued collaboration of palliative care and bioethics can be expected to strengthen their individual efforts and enrich their joint contribution to health care.

References

Alpers. A. (1998). Criminal act or palliative care? Prosecutions involving the care of the dying. *The Journal of Law, Medicine & Ethics.* 26(4):308-331.

Arnold, R.M. (2002). A roles by any other name. *Journal of Palliative Medicine.* 5(6):807-817.

Back, A.L. and Arnold, R.M. (2005). Dealing with conflict in caring for the seriously ill: "It was just out of the question." *Journal of the American Medical Association.* 293(11):1374-1381.

Beauchamp, T.L. and Childress, J.F. (2001). *Principles of Biomedical Ethics, Fifth Edition.* Oxford University Press, New York.

Blustein, J., Post, L.F., and Dubler, N.N. (2004). Holding health care organizations norally accountable. *Keynotes on Health Care.* 35(3):1-8.

Blustein, J., Post, L.F., and Dubler, N.N. (2002). *Ethics for Health Care Organizations: Theory, Case Studies, and Tools.* United Hospital Fund, New York.

Bretscher, M.E. and Creagan, E.T. (1997). Understanding suffering: What palliative medicine teaches us. *Mayo Clinic Proceedings.* 72(8):785-787.

Brumley, R.D. (2002). Future of end-of-life care: The managed care organization perspective. *Journal of Palliative Medicine.* 5(2):263-270.

Calderone, K.L. (1990). The influence of gender on the frequency of pain and sedative medication administered to post-operative patients. *Sex Roles.* 23(11/12):713-725.

Christakis, N.A. (1998). Attitude and self-reported practice regarding prognostication in a national sample of internists. *Archives of Internal Medicine.* 158(21):2389-2395.

Cleeland, C.S., Gonin, R., Hatfield, A.K., Edmonson, J.H., Blum, R.H., Stewart, J.A., and Pandya, K.J. (1994). Pain and its treatment in outpatients with metastatic cancer. *New England Journal of Medicine.* 330(9):592-596.

Cleeland, C.S., Gonin, R., Baez, L., Loehrer, P., and Pandya, K.J. (1997). Pain and treatment of pain in minority patients with cancer. *Annals of Internal Medicine.* 127(9):813-816.

Davis, M.P., Walsh, D., LeGrand, S.B., and Lagman, R. (2002). End-of-life care: The death of palliative medicine? *Journal of Palliative Medicine.* 5(6):813-814.

Desbiens N.A., Wu, A.W., Broste, S.K., Wenger, N.S., Connors, A.F., Lynn, J., Yasui, Y., Phillips, R.S., and Fulkerson, W. (1996). Pain and satisfaction with pain control in seriously ill hospitalized adults: Findings from the SUPPORT research investigations. *Journal of the American Medical Association.* 24(12):1953-1961.

Dubler, N.N. and Liebman, C.B. (2004). *Bioethics Mediation: A Guide to Shaping Shared Solutions.* United Hospital Fund, New York.

Epstein, A.M. and Ayanian, J.Z. (2001). Editorial: Racial disparities in medical care. *New England Journal of Medicine.* 344(19):1471-1473.

Fischer, G.S., Tulsky, J.A., Rose, M.R., Siminoff, L.A., and Arnold, R.M. (1998). Patient knowledge and physician predictions of treatment preferences after discussion of advance directives. *Journal of General Internal Medicine.* 13(7):447-454.

Foley, K.M. (1995). Misconceptions and controversies regarding the use of opioids in cancer pain. *Anti-Cancer Drugs.* 6(Supp3):4-13.

Freeman, H.P. and Payne, R. (2000). Racial injustice in health care. *New England Journal of Medicine.* 342(14):1045-1047.

Gillick, M.R. (2004). Advance care planning. *New England Journal of Medicine* 350(1):7-8.

Gross, M.D. (1998). What do patients express as their preferences in advance directives? *Archives of Internal Medicine.* 158(4):363-365.

Hammes, B.J. and Rooney, B.L. (1998). Death and end-of-life planning in one Midwestern community. *Archives of Internal Medicine.* 158(4):383-390.

Jecker, N.S., Carrese, J.A., and Pearlman, R.A. (1995). Caring for patients in cross-cultural settings. *Hastings Center Report.* 25(1):6-14.

Lemeshow, S., Teres, D., Klar, J., Avrunin, J.S., Gehlbach, S.H., and Rapoport, J. (1993). Mortality Probability Models (MPM II) based on an international cohort of intensive care until patients. *Journal of the American Medical Association.* 270(20):2478-2486.

Lo, B. and Steinbrook, R. (2004). Resuscitating advance directives. *Archives of Internal Medicine.* 164(14):1501-1506.

Loewy, E.H. (1998). Ethical considerations in executing and implementing advance directives. *Archives of Internal Medicine.* 158(4):321-24.

Luce, J.M. (1995). Physicians do not have a responsibility to provide futile or unreasonable care if a patient or family insists. *Critical Care Medicine.* 23(4):760-766.

Morrison, R.S., Wallenstein, S., Natale, D.K., Senzel, R.S., and Huang, L.L. (2000). "We don't carry that"—Failure of pharmacies in predominantly nonwhite neighborhoods to stock opioid analgesics. *New England Journal of Medicine.* 342(14):1023-1026.

Morrison, R.S., Zayas, L.H., Mulvihill, M., Baskin, S.A., and Meier, D.E. (1998). Barriers to completion of health care proxies: An examination of ethnic differences. *Archives of Internal Medicine.* 158(22):2493-2497.

Morrison, R.S., Olson, E., Mertz, K.R., and Meier, D.E. (1995). The inaccessibility of advance directives on transfer from abulatory to acute care settings. *Journal of the American Medical Association.* 374(6):478-482.

Ng, B., Dimsdale, J.E., Rollnik, J.D., and Shapiro, J. (1996). The effect of ethnicity on prescriptions for patient-controlled analgesia for post-operative pain. *Pain.* 66:9-12.

O'Mahony, S., McHugh, M., Zallman, L., and Selwyn, P. (2003). Ventilator withdrawal: Procedures and outcomes. Report of a collaboration between a critical care division and a palliative care service. *Journal of Pain and Symptom Management.* 26(4):954-960.

Pellegrino, E.D. (1992). Intersections of Western biomedical ethics and world culture. *Cambridge Quarterly of Healthcare Ethics.* Summer 1(3):191-6.

Pellegrino, E.D., Mazzarella, P., and Corsi, P. (eds), *Transcultural Demensions in Medical Ethics.* University Publishing Group, Inc., Frederick, MD.

Pellegrino, E.S. (1993). Patient and physician autonomy: Conflicting rights and obligations in the patient-physician relationship. *Journal of Contemporary Health Law and Policy.* 10:47-86.

Phillips, R.S., Hamel, M.B., Teno, J.M., Bellamy, P., Broste, S.K., Califf, R.M., Vidailet, H., Davis, R.B., Muhlbaier, L.H., Connors, A.F., Lynn, J., and Goldman, L., for the SUPPORT Investigators. (1996). Race, resource use, and survival in seriously ill hospitalized adults. *Journal of General Internal Medicine.* 11(7):387-396.

Post, L.F., Blustein, J., and Dubler, N.N. (2007). *Handbook for Health Care Ethics Committees.* The Johns Hopkins University Press, Baltimore.

Post, L.F. (2006). Living wills and durable powers of attorney. In Schulz, R., Noelker, L.S., Rockwood, K., Sprott, R.L. (eds.) The Encyclopedia of Aging, 4th ed. New York: Springer Publishing Company.

Post, L.F. (2003). Clinical consultation: The search for resolution at the intersection of medicine, law, and ethics. *HEC Forum.* 15(4):338-351.

Post, L.F., Blustein, J., Gordon, E., and Dubler, N.N. (1996). Pain: Ethics, culture and informed consent to relief. *Journal of Law, Medicine & Ethics.* 24:348-359.

Post, L.F. and Dubler, N.N. (1997). Palliative care: A bioethical definition, principles, and clinical guidelines. *Bioethics Forum.* 13(3):17-24.

Prendergast, T.J. (2001). Advance care planning: Pitfalls, progress, promise. *Critical Care Medicine.* 29(2) Supplement, N34-N39.

Smith, T.J., Coyne, P., Cassel, B., Penberthy, L., Hopson, A., and Hager, M.A. (2003). A high-volume specialist palliative care unit and team may reduce in-hospital end-of-life care costs. *Journal of Palliative Medicine.* 6(5):699-705.

Sprung, C.L., Eidelman, L.A., and Steinberg, A. (1995). Is the physician's duty to the individual patient or to society? *Critical Care Medicine.* 23(4):618-620.

SUPPORT Principal Investigators. (1995). A controlled trial to improve care for seriously ill hospitalized patients: The study to understand prognoses and preferences for outcomes and risks of treatments (SUPPORT). *Journal of the American Medical Association.* 274:1591-1598.

Teno, J.M., Stevens, M., Spernak, S., and Lynn, J. (1998). Role of written advance directives in decision making: Insights from qualitative and quantitative data. *Journal of General Internal Medicine.* 13(7):439-446.

Todd, K.H., Deaton C., D'Adamo, A.P., Goe, L. (2000). Ethnicity and analgesic practice. *Annals of Emergency Medicine.* 35(1):11-16.

Todd, K.H., Lee, T., and Hoffman, J.R. (1994). The effect of ethnicity on physician estimates of pain severity in patients with isolated extremity trauma. *Journal of the American Medical Association.* 271(12):925-928.

Todd, K.H., Samaroo, N., and Hoffman, J.R. (1993). Ethnicity as a risk factor for inadequate emergency department analgesia. *Journal of the American Medical Association.* 269(12):1537-1539.

Vacco v. Quill, 521 U.S. 793 (1997).

Walsh, D., Gombeski, W.R., Goldstein, P., Hayes, D., and Armour, M. (1994). Managing a palliative oncology program: The role of a business plan. *Journal of Pain and Symptom Management.* 9(2):109-118.

Washington v. Glucksberg, 521 U.S. 702 (1997).

Wissow, L.S., Belote, A., Kramer, W., Compton-Phillips, A., Kritzler, R., and Weiner, J.P. (2004). Promoting advance directives among elderly primary care patients. *Journal of General Internal Medicine.* 19(9):944-951.

Wolf, S.H. (2004). Society's choice: The tradeoff between efficacy and equity and the lives at stake. *American Journal of Preventive Medicine.* 27(1):49-56.

Youngner, S.J. (1988). Who defines futility? *Journal of the American Medical Association.* 260(14):2094-2095.

Zenz, M. (1991). Morphine myths: Sedation, tolerance, addiction. *Postgraduate Medicine Journal.* 67(Supp. 2):S100-S102.

Index

Printed in the United States
77163LV00001B/67-75